Brice Kevin KOLLO NZIMA

Determinants of self-medication with NSAIDs in Abidjan

Brice Kevin KOLLO NZIMA

Determinants of self-medication with NSAIDs in Abidjan

ScienciaScripts

Imprint

Any brand names and product names mentioned in this book are subject to trademark, brand or patent protection and are trademarks or registered trademarks of their respective holders. The use of brand names, product names, common names, trade names, product descriptions etc. even without a particular marking in this work is in no way to be construed to mean that such names may be regarded as unrestricted in respect of trademark and brand protection legislation and could thus be used by anyone.

Cover image: www.ingimage.com

This book is a translation from the original published under ISBN 978-620-6-71149-0.

Publisher:
Sciencia Scripts
is a trademark of
Dodo Books Indian Ocean Ltd. and OmniScriptum S.R.L publishing group

120 High Road, East Finchley, London, N2 9ED, United Kingdom
Str. Armeneasca 28/1, office 1, Chisinau MD-2012, Republic of Moldova, Europe
Printed at: see last page
ISBN: 978-620-8-07794-5

Contents

Visit
lord god almighty

Acknowledgements

TO ALMIGHTY GOD,

With all my heart Father, I give you thanks for all the knowledge I have acquired and for your presence in my life. Thank You Father, My rock, my soul never forgets any of Your blessings.

To my grandfather, Théodore ANDOSEH

You are my role model, and it's thanks to you that I have specialised in rheumatology, especially in Côte d'Ivoire.

To my dear parents, Bernadette and Jacques NZIMA

You made me what I am today. Thank you so much for your constant presence. May the Lord keep you with us for a long time so that you can enjoy the fruits of your efforts.

To my dear spiritual parents, Neuly and Joseph NGANDEU

Thank you so much for your presence in my life and your invaluable advice. May the Lord keep you with us for a long time.

To my beloved, Evelyne NZIMA,

You are the one who gives meaning to the love in my life, the strength that gives me hope, the reason for my perseverance. This work, which is also yours, is the fruit of your hardships, of all your sacrifices, of your invaluable support. Please accept my deepest gratitude. May God grant us the grace of happiness.

To my sister and younger brothers, Naomi, Donald and Emmanuel

For all your contributions to the success of this adventure.

To Mother Madeleine KOFFI,

Thank you for welcoming me to Côte d'Ivoire over the last 4 years.

To my friend Sostelle Konné,

You have made my stay easier by your presence among those I have left behind.

To my spiritual children,

Thank you for being with me and making me happy.

To my parents-in-law, Clotilde and Jean Claude Awala

Please accept my deepest gratitude.

To my brothers and sisters in the faith,

Thank you for your prayers.

To all my fellow graduates: Drs BISSEH Vanessa, Eric DANGUI, Enoch KOFFI, Guilène KLOKOUIE, Vilette NKWUITCHOUA, Irène MENDO, Inès SIMO,

For everything we've been through together. A brilliant career to you all!

To all our other DES colleagues,

Thank you for this great collaboration.

To our teacher in Cameroon, Professor Madeleine NGANDEU

Thanks for the support and advice

To all the rheumatologists who contributed to our training, in particular Doctors Nina KPAMI, Yaya COULIBALY, Aboubacar BAMBA, Abidou COULIBALY, Franck BROU, Sandrine WABO, Raphaël KOUASSI, Alexis YOBOUE and Alaine KONAN,

Thank you for your availability.

To all the staff of the rheumatology department of the CHU de Cocody

Thank you for your cooperation and support.

To all those who have contributed in any way to the success of this adventure

Many thanks.

To the Chairman of the Jury, Professor Edmond ETI

It is a great honour for you to chair the jury for our dissertation defence. We are convinced that your advice and recommendations will help us to perfect this work.

Thank you, dear Master, for the training and all the time you gave us. Through these tributes, please accept the expression of our great admiration and the testimony of our sincere respect for you. Distinguished and respectful tributes!

To jury member MCA Mermoz DJAHA,

You guided us, gave us direction and supported us throughout the course. Your simplicity and humility, as well as your selflessness, have always impressed us. You agreed to take the time to judge this work. Your analyses will help to improve it. We can't find the right words to thank you, dear Master, but please accept the expression of our deepest gratitude. Respectful tributes!

To our thesis supervisor, Professor Mohamed DIOMANDE

Dear Master, how can I thank you in so few words for everything you have done since the beginning of our training. The privilege you have given us by agreeing to direct this work gives us the opportunity to express our gratitude. With regular spontaneity, you have opened your doors to us. Please find here, dear Master, the expression of our deepest gratitude. Respectful homage!

To Professor Marcel KOUAKOU NZUE,

For all the knowledge you have passed on. Respectful tributes!

To our Master, Professor Félix Jean-Claude DABOIKO,

We admire the immensity of your knowledge. Please find here, dear Master, the testimony of our greatest respect. Respectful homage!

To our Master, MCA Baly OUATTARA,

We have always marvelled at your great scientific mind. This is the moment to thank you sincerely for all the lessons you have taught us. Please find here the expression of our great admiration. Respectful tributes!

To our Master, Professor Mariam GBANE,

Our gratitude for your constant presence at our side and your humility. Your scientific rigour, your availability and your modesty command respect and inspire admiration. Your methodical teaching will serve us well for the rest of our lives. Respectful tributes!

Introduction

Non-steroidal anti-inflammatory drugs (NSAIDs) are one of the most widely used therapeutic classes in the world [1]. More than 300 million people worldwide take NSAIDs, and 30 million patients take NSAIDs on a daily basis [2,3]. Their analgesic, antipyretic and anti-inflammatory properties explain why they are widely used for symptomatic purposes, in particular to relieve or even prevent pain [4-8]. Their potential toxicity is all the greater when the people affected by their use include the elderly, people at risk of polymedication or people with other co-morbidities [9]. Misuse of NSAIDs will inexorably lead to damage to the user (peptic ulcer, haemorrhage, arterial hypertension, renal failure, etc.) [2,9]. This misuse comes under the heading of self-medication, which, according to the WHO, "consists in the fact that an individual resorts to a medicine, on his own initiative or that of a relative, with the aim of treating an ailment or symptom that he has identified himself, without having recourse to a health professional"; it can involve both modern and traditional medicine [10]. It is a worldwide phenomenon and therefore a public health problem [2,11-13]. Its prevalence has risen sharply worldwide, and according to Gora et al, up to 80% of all medicines are bought without a prescription in developing countries [14]. More than 50% of all medicines prescribed, dispensed or sold are currently used inappropriately [15,16]. This has the above-mentioned consequences. Self-medication with NSAIDs should therefore be avoided. The prevalence of self-medication in Africa ranged from 27.16% to 91.4% [17,18]. The motivations, harms and drugs involved in self-medication have been studied [17,19-24]. In the literature, the reasons for self-medication were: the high cost of treating patients in health facilities, low purchasing power, a shortage of health infrastructure and staff, the trivialisation of certain diseases, the complicity of some pharmacy salespeople who do not respect the rules for dispensing medicines, and the lack of information and awareness of the risks associated with misuse of medicines [19,25-27]. In our context, few related studies have been carried out [27-29], and to our knowledge there are none on self-medication with NSAIDs. A study looking at factors influencing the use of street medicines identified the following factors: profession and socio-economic level [27]. Thus, our general objective was to identify the factors determining the practice of self-medication with NSAIDs among our patients in order to positively influence this practice and consequently abandon it.

The specific objectives were :

- Determine the hospital frequency of self-medication with NSAIDs
- Describe the sociodemographic, clinical and therapeutic aspects of patients self-medicating with NSAIDs

-    To investigate the influence of socio-demographic and clinical factors on patients' self-medication with NSAIDs.

Chapter 1

General

1. NON-STEROIDAL ANTI-INFLAMMATORY DRUGS

I-1. DEFINITION [30-32]

NSAIDs are a widely used therapeutic class due to their antipyretic, analgesic and anti-inflammatory properties. They are used in a wide range of indications, including osteo-muscular pain, rheumatological conditions, renal colic and traumatology.

NSAIDs have a purely symptomatic action, acting on the pathophysiology of inflammation, without acting on its aetiology, which must be treated separately. They are among the most frequently prescribed drugs in the world (accounting for 4.5% of drug consumption in industrialised countries), with a significant proportion also being self-medicated. Both their efficacy and their main side-effects are linked to their main mechanism of action, which is the inhibition of cyclooxygenases.

I-2. MECHANISM OF ACTION [33-35]

The discovery of the principal mechanism of action of NSAIDs is due to the work of **Vane**, **Samuelson and Bergstrom** (1971). The mechanism of action of NSAIDs involves reducing the production of prostanoids by inhibiting an enzyme, cyclooxygenase (Cox). Prostanoids (prostaglandins D2, E2, F2, prostacyclin, thromboxane A2) are eicosanoids with a purely local action. However, their almost ubiquitous distribution means that they are involved in many physiological and pathological processes. They are synthesised from arachidonic acid (itself derived from membrane phospholipids) by Cox, of which there are two isoenzymes:

■ Cox-1, present in constitutive form in almost all tissues, catalyses the formation of prostaglandins involved in the cytoprotection of the gastric mucosa and the preservation of renal function, as well as the production of thromboxane A2 (TxA2, a vasoconstrictor and proaggregant) by platelets.

NSAIDs (gastric toxicity, reduced renal blood flow and anti-platelet aggregation effect).

■ Cox-2, which is essentially an isoenzyme that is inducible in inflammatory states, leads to the release of prostaglandins that have a pathological role (fever, pain, inflammation, cell proliferation), but also a beneficial role in various processes (healing, renal function, ovulation, etc.) and govern the synthesis of prostacyclin (PGI2), a vasodilator and antiaggregant, by endothelial cells. Its inhibition is responsible for the pharmacodynamic effects of NSAIDs (anti-inflammatory effect as well as analgesic and antipyretic effects).

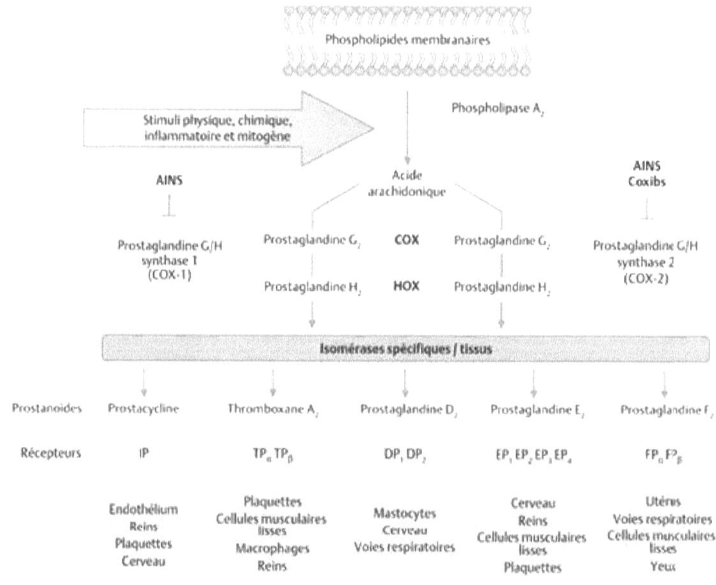

Figure 1: Metabolism of arachidonic acid and synthesis of prostanoids [34].

I-3. PHARMACOKINETICS [35]

I-3-1. Reductions

NSAIDs are weak lipophilic acids: rapid and almost complete resorption. Peak plasma levels are reached in 30 minutes to 2 hours for standard forms. Apart from specific situations, obtaining the peak more quickly by using injectable forms does not increase their efficacy. Treatment by parenteral route is only rarely justified and must be limited in time.

I-3-2. Broadcasting

Protein binding is high (>90%) with a risk of therapeutic interaction and risk of displacement with an increase in the free fraction of either the NSAID or its competitor. Risk of toxicity from acute overdose. NSAIDs diffuse well into tissue and synovial fluid. It crosses the foeto-placental barrier, the blood-brain barrier and passes very slightly into breast milk.

I-3-3. Metabolism and elimination

Most NSAIDs are metabolised in the liver, leading to the formation of inactive metabolites, which are eliminated in the kidneys (60%) and faeces, with an enterohepatic cycle (40%).

I-3-4. Routes of administration

I-3-4-1. General pathways [34]

These routes all carry the same risks, to which specific local complications are sometimes added:

■ oral route: this is the preferred route, especially as bioavailability is excellent (>90%);

■ rectal route: suppositories are absorbed more irregularly than oral forms;

■ intramuscular route: this route is particularly useful when oral administration is not possible, in an emergency situation, due to its rapid onset of action. In practice, its use should be limited to 48 to 72 hours, only if other routes of administration are not possible;

■ intravenous route: according to the AMM, this route is reserved for specific indications such as the treatment of postoperative pain or the treatment of attacks of renal colic. It should not be continued for more than 72 hours.

I-3-4-2. Local route [34]

Applications of NSAID gel or ointment may be sufficient to relieve pain associated with a minor sprain, contusion, tendonitis or osteoarthritis of small joints. These forms of NSAID may cause local hypersensitivity reactions, or even undesirable effects if used for a long time, due to the low systemic absorption of the NSAID.

I-4. THERAPEUTIC PROPERTIES

I-4-1. Antipyretic action [34]

NSAIDs reduce fever, whatever its origin (infectious, inflammatory or neoplastic), by inhibiting the synthesis of PGE2, induced by the action of IL-1 on the hypothalamic thermoregulatory centre. They do not induce hypothermia in normal subjects.

I-4-2. Analgesic action [34]

NSAIDs are peripheral analgesics. They act within the algogenic focus, where prostaglandins play an etiopathogenic role in nociception.

I-4-3. Anti-inflammatory action [34,35].

NSAIDs act above all on the early, vascular component of inflammation (inhibition of certain functions such as chemotaxis, cell adhesion and phagocytosis) responsible for the classic "pain, redness, heat, tumour" tetrad. It is used in acute microcrystalline attacks (gout, chondrocalcinosis), abarticular pathologies, spinal and radicular pathologies and chronic inflammatory rheumatism (rheumatoid arthritis and spondyloarthropathy).

I-4-4. Anti-platelet aggregation action [33,34,36].

It is caused by all NSAIDs, but especially acetylsalicylic acid, whose action on cyclooxygenase is irreversible. The cyclooxygenase pathway leads to the formation of TXA2, a powerful aggregating and vasoconstrictive agent. Platelets do not contain COX-2 but only COX-1. Platelet TXA2 can therefore only be derived from COX-1 activity. Acetylsalicylic acid is a preferential inhibitor of COX-1, but "low-dose" acetylsalicylic acid is a selective inhibitor of COX-1. Acetylsalicylic acid acts on COX, irreversibly preventing the formation of PGG2. None of the other NSAIDs acts by this particular mechanism and all are reversible inhibitors. Since acetylsalicylic acid has a greater affinity (150 to 200 times) for COX-1 than for COX-2, it selectively and durably inhibits (at low doses) platelet COX-1, resulting in total and irreversible inhibition of TXA2 synthesis. This irreversible blockade lasts for the entire lifespan of the platelets (around 7 days) because they are unable to synthesise COX de novo. A low dose of acetylsalicylic acid is sufficient to block more than 95% of platelet TXA2 production, but daily administration is still necessary because significant amounts of TXA2 are synthesised once 10-15% of platelets have been reconstituted. On the other hand, a single daily dose of acetylsalicylic acid does not significantly inhibit PGI2 synthesis because the interval between the 2 doses allows the endothelial cell to restore COX-1 activity without altering COX-2-dependent PGI2 production. Conventional "non-selective" NSAIDs, which are reversible inhibitors of platelet COX-1, can, in theory, inhibit platelet aggregation, but only during the period when their serum concentration is sufficient. It is likely that the superior cardioprotective effect of "low dose" acetylsalicylic acid compared with other NSAIDs is linked to this pharmacological difference. Recent NSAIDs known as selective COX-2 inhibitors inhibit COX-2 without inhibiting platelet COX-1, at all therapeutic concentrations. The collateral effect of selective COX-2 inhibitors is therefore the absence of inhibition of platelet COX-1 and, consequently, the absence of an anti-platelet aggregation effect. It therefore seems logical to maintain the use of "low-dose" acetylsalicylic acid when coxib is taken concomitantly by a patient at cardiovascular risk. The antiaggregant effect of acetylsalicylic acid requires only low doses (<300 mg/d) and persists for around a week after treatment is stopped.

I-5. CLASSIFICATION

I-5-1. According to the chemical classification [33,34]

NSAIDs are compounds, some of which have structural similarities. They can therefore be classified by chemical family.

Table I: chemical family of NSAIDs [34].

Chemical family		DCI
Salicylates		Acetylsalicylic acid Lysine acetylsalicylate Carbasalate calcium
Arlycarboxylic	Propionics	Tiaprofenic acid Fenoprofen Flurbiprofen Ibuprofen Ketoprofen Naproxen sodium Alminoprofen
	Phenylacetates	Etodolac Diclofenac Aceclofenac
Fenamates		Niflumic acid
Indolines		Indomethacin
		Sulindac
Oxicams		Meloxicam
		Piroxicam
		Tenoxicam
Sulfonalidine		Nimesulin
Pyrazoles		Phenylbutazone
Coxibs		Celecoxib
		Etoricoxib

I-5-2. According to the respective action of NSAIDs [33,34]

The duality of cyclooxygenase (COX) leads to a distinction being made between :

■ selective COX-1 inhibitors: represented by low-dose acetylsalicylic acid (300 mg per day or less), used as an antiaggregant for anti-thrombotic purposes, but also indomethacin and piroxicam ;

■ non-selective COX inhibitors, all of which inhibit Cox-2 and Cox-1 at therapeutic doses; the majority of "classic NSAIDs

■ Preferential COX-2 inhibitors: because of their ability to inhibit COX-1, but only for the highest recommended doses (meloxicam; nimesulide).

■ Selective COX-2 inhibitors (Coxibs): celecoxib, parecoxib, which differ from the above in that they have a lower ulcerogenic risk and no anti-platelet effect.

I-5-3. Depending on the generation of NSAIDs [33]

This classification has the merit of clarifying the availability of NSAIDs at different times.

<u>**Table II**</u>: Classification of NSAIDs by generation [33].

	Groups	DCI	Speciality name
1ere generation (1950-1960)	Salicylates	Acetylsalicylic acid	Aspirin
	Pyrazoles	Phenylbutazone	Butazolidine
	Indolent	Indomethacin	Indocid
	Fenamates	Niflumic acid	Nifluril
2e generation (1970-1980)	Arylpropionics	Ibuprofen	Brufen
	Arylacetic	Diclofenac	Voltarene
	Oxicams	Piroxicam	Feldène
3e generation (1990-2000)	Sulfonalidine	Nimesulide	Nexen
	Oxicams	Meloxicam	Mobic
4e generation (2000-2010)	Coxib	Rofecoxib	Vioxx
		Celecoxib	Celebrex
		Paracecoxib	Dynasta
		Etoricoxib	Arcoxia

I-5-4. According to the half-life [34]

<u>**Table III**</u>: Classification of the main NSAIDs according to their duration of action [34].

	DCI
Short half-life (< 6 hours)	Ketoprofen Ibuprofen Furbiprofen Niflumic acid Tiaprofenic acid Alminoprofen Diclofenac
Intermediate half-life	Sulindac Naproxen Naproxen sodium Étodolac Meloxicam
Long half-life (< 24 hours)	Piroxicam Tenoxicam Piroxicam β-cyclodextrin
Prolonged release (>24 hours)	Indomethacin Ketoprofen Dicolfenac

NB: Some NSAIDs may share a short, intermediate, long or even prolonged half-life.

Example: Diclofenac 50 mg (short half-life)

Diclofenac 75mg (intermediate half-life)

Diclofenac 100 mg LP (Extended Release)

I-6-. INDICATIONS AND CONTRAINDICATIONS

I-6.1 Indications [34,37,38].

Despite their pharmacological similarities, not all NSAIDs have the same indications. This is due to differences in their benefit/risk ratio and in the clinical trials carried out to obtain their marketing authorisation. It is therefore necessary to consult the *Vidal* dictionary to find out the exact wording of the recognised indications for each product. Broadly speaking, there are three types of NSAID:

■ List I NSAIDs, indole derivatives (indomethacin and sulindac), certain arylcarboxylics (diclofenac suppository, diclofenac combined with misoprostol, nabumetone, etc.), oxicam derivatives (piroxicam, tenoxicam and meloxicam) and nimesulide.), oxicam derivatives (piroxicam, tenoxicam and meloxicam) and nimesulide: generally intended for all painful or disabling rheumatological conditions (acute or chronic inflammatory rheumatism, osteoarthritis, tendonitis, bursitis, acute radiculalgia);

■ AINS on list II, arylcarboxylic derivatives (naproxen, etodalac, tiaprofenic acid, ketoprofen, alminoprofen, flirbuprofen, ibuprofen, aceclofenac, diclofenac) and fenamates (niflumic acid, morniflumate): which may be authorised in the above indications and in traumatology (sprains), ENT and stomatology (sinusitis, otitis, dental pain), gynaecology (primary dysmenorrhoea, functional menorrhagia), urology (renal colic) and febrile conditions;

■ Non-listed MEDICINES: low-dose MEDICINES (acetylsalicylic acid, ibuprofen) that do not require a prescription and are used for the symptomatic treatment of painful or febrile conditions.

I-6-2. Contraindications [9,34]

Table IV: List of contraindications for NSAIDs [9,34].

All NSAIDs		- Active peptic ulcer, - History of peptic ulcer or recurrent haemorrhage (at least 2 documented episodes), - Severe hepatocellular insufficiency, - History of digestive bleeding or perforation on NSAIDs - Severe cardiac insufficiency, - Severe renal insufficiency.
Additional contraindications	Coxibs Diclofenac	- Proven ischaemic heart disease, - Peripheral arterial disease, - Previous cerebrovascular accident (including transient ischaemic attack).
	Etoricoxib	- Uncontrolled hypertension
Pregnancy	Coxibs	- Throughout pregnancy
	Other NSAIDs	- From the beginning of the 6th month of

		pregnancy (24 weeks of amenorrhoea)

I-6-3. Prescription procedures

I-6-3-1. Personalised assessment of the benefit/risk ratio [34].

It must take into account the indication, the patient's condition, co-morbidities and the drugs being taken. In practice, NSAIDs should only be used for inflammatory rheumatism, especially spondyloarthritis. In all other potential indications, NSAIDs appear to be an alternative to other analgesics when the latter are ineffective, contraindicated or poorly tolerated. Paracetamol remains the first-line analgesic for most pain syndromes of moderate intensity, particularly in the elderly. Similarly, it is often preferable to use a low-dose oral corticosteroid in rheumatoid arthritis in patients at risk of digestive or renal damage from NSAIDs. If an NSAID fails at the recommended dosage, another compound should be tried because of the individual variability in response to a given NSAID. In all cases, the minimum useful dose should be used, starting with medium or even low doses, particularly in degenerative rheumatism and in elderly patients, since the main adverse effects of NSAIDs are dose-dependent. As these drugs are purely symptomatic, treatment should be discontinued during periods of remission.

■ **Children and the elderly** [39,40]

Medicines are prescribed differently for adults, children and the elderly. Children under the age of 15 do not metabolise medicines in the same way as adults. People over 65 have kidney and liver functions that function less well. Medicines are therefore less well metabolised and/or eliminated. The choice of medicine, dosage and duration of prescription will depend on the patient's age. To treat pain and/or fever in children under the age of 15, only 5 NSAIDs are currently authorised in France: ibuprofen, ketoprofen, mefenamic acid, niflumic acid and tiaprofenic acid.

■ **Pregnancy and breastfeeding** [39,41].

NSAIDs should be avoided because of the harmful effects they can have on the embryo, foetus and mother. This applies to all routes of administration, including the cutaneous route. Eye drops, however, can be used during pregnancy due to the small quantities used. When breast-feeding, NSAIDs should be avoided because these molecules can pass into breast milk. As they act on prostaglandins, this will cause numerous side effects. Reye's syndrome may occur if a breast-feeding mother takes acetylsalicylic acid with a child suffering from a viral pathology (chickenpox, influenza, measles, rubella).

I-7. DRUG INTERACTIONS [9]

I-7-1. Major interactions

■ Anticoagulant: increased risk of haemorrhage.

■ piroxicam and acetylsalicylic acid in anti-inflammatory doses: contraindicated combination

■ other NSAIDs: combination not recommended. When this combination is essential, it requires close clinical and even biological monitoring.

■ Methotrexate: increased haematological toxicity of methotrexate due to displacement of methotrexate from its plasma protein binding.

■ Hypoglycaemic sulphonamides: increase in the hypoglycaemic effect of sulphonamides by displacement of the oral antidiabetic from its plasma protein binding.

■ Lithium: risk of lithium overdose due to reduced renal elimination of lithium. This leads to effects such as neuropsychological disorders, memory disorders, endocrine disorders, skin disorders, cardiac disorders and haematological disorders.

■ Anti-platelet agents: increased risk of digestive haemorrhage. Patients on anti-platelet acetylsalicylic acid should be warned of the risks of self-medication with acetylsalicylic acid or another NSAID.

I-7-2. Average interactions

■ Diuretics: by modifying renal haemodynamics, NSAIDs alter the action of diuretics. This results in a reduction in their efficacy and therefore a reduction in the antihypertensive effect, especially as NSAIDs tend to induce fluid retention. Risk of acute renal failure in patients at risk (elderly and/or dehydrated patients).

■ Anti-hypertensives: Converting enzyme inhibitor (CEI), angiotensin II receptor antagonist (ARB II). Risk of acute renal failure in patients at risk (elderly and/or dehydrated patients).

■ Digitalis: modification of renal excretion by digitalis increases digoxin levels and therefore the risk of cardiac toxicity from digitalis.

■ Probenicide: It is a uricosuric by reducing the tubular reabsorption of urates used in the basic treatment of gout and more generally in the management of symptomatic hyperuricemia. Its effect disappears in cases of renal insufficiency with a creatinine clearance value of less than 80ml/min, hence the interaction with NSAIDs.

■ Phenytoin: risk of phenytoin overload due to displacement of phenytoin from its plasma protein binding.

I-8. MAIN UNDESIRABLE EFFECTS

Virtually all NSAIDs are associated with the same complications. However, the incidence of a given adverse reaction depends on the nature of the NSAID and often its dosage, as well as the patient's condition and associated medications [34].

I-8-1. Digestive effects [2,34,42-46].

These are the most common (15-25%), with suppression of the synthesis of the prostaglandins PGE2 and PGI2, through inhibition of cyclooxygenases, leading to a reduction in the blood supply to the mucous membrane and its secretion of bicarbonate. These two mechanisms make the gastrointestinal mucosa more vulnerable to the deleterious effects of gastric acid or inflammation. They can develop on healthy intestinal mucosa or complicate the evolution of pre-existing conditions.

■ functional upper digestive symptoms (dyspepsia, gastralgia, nausea): frequent and rapidly resolved when the product is stopped. They are poorly correlated with lesions of the gastroduodenal mucosa;

■ gastroduodenal ulcers: more frequent with conventional NSAIDs than with coxibs, and asymptomatic in half of cases. Complications of ulcers: digestive haemorrhage, perforation, sometimes occurring early, occur at a rate of 2 to 4% patient-years with conventional NSAIDs. These complications occur mainly in patients with risk factors. This risk is approximately half as high with coxibs, although this advantage is lost when the patient is simultaneously taking acetylsalicylic acid for anti-thrombotic purposes.

■ Intestinal digestive complications: ulceration of the small intestine and colon, often unrecognised, sometimes with complications (perforation, haemorrhage, anaemia). NSAIDs are thought to encourage diverticulitis flare-ups in patients with diverticulosis.

Table V: Risk factors for serious digestive complications on NSAIDs [34].

• Elderly: age > 65 years.
• History of peptic ulcer or upper digestive haemorrhage or *Helicobacter pylori* infection.
• Severe co-morbidities.
• NSAIDs used in high doses or a combination of two NSAIDs.
• Co-prescription of aspirin (even in low doses for platelet anti-aggregation), anti-coagulants, platelet anti-aggregants and corticoids.
• Inflammatory disease (e.g. rheumatoid arthritis).

Where there is a risk factor, the co-prescription of a half-dose proton pump inhibitor (PPI) should be systematic with the prescription of an NSAID.

I-8-2. Renal effects [2,34,47-49].

The most common are early-onset, dose-dependent and the result of renal Cox inhibition.

- Acute renal failure (ARF): ARF tends to occur in elderly patients or patients with hypovolaemia. The risk factors are :
- treatment with diuretics, conversion enzyme inhibitors or angiotensin II antagonists;
- dehydration;
- de-sodified diet;
- heart failure.

■ Hypertension due to fluid retention: Blood pressure must be monitored during prolonged treatment.

■ Chronic renal failure: Chronic renal failure due to chronic tubulointerstitial nephropathy may occur with long-term treatment with NSAIDs. It is necessary to monitor glomerular filtration rate during prolonged treatment.

I-8-3. Cardiovascular effects [2,34,50].

■ **Arterial thrombotic risk**

The thrombotic effects (myocardial infarction and stroke) of Cox-2 inhibitors are low (3 to 4 events per 1000 patient-years), although this risk has been confirmed in numerous studies. However, all NSAIDs, especially those used in high doses, may be responsible for arterial thrombosis, with a greater risk for coxibs and diclofenac, and to a lesser extent Ibuprofen, according to data from meta-analyses of randomised trials. With naproxen, the risk appears to be lower. Current data suggest that this risk exists even with short-term prescriptions.

■ **Heart failure**

Heart failure associated with NSAIDs is more likely in patients with a history of any form of heart disease. The use of NSAIDs in elderly patients taking diuretics is associated with twice the risk of hospitalisation for heart failure.

■ **Risk of thromboembolic events**

Prescription of NSAIDs appears to be associated with an increased relative risk of thromboembolic events (deep vein thrombosis and pulmonary embolism).

I-8-4. Gynaeco-obstetrical effects [2,9,34,39,41].

By inhibiting Cox-2, NSAIDs have a tocolytic effect. They expose the foetus to premature closure of the ductus arteriosus and renal failure from the sixth month of pregnancy. During pregnancy, the level of PGF2α, synthesised in the uterus, increases until it reaches a certain concentration, triggering delivery. When an NSAID is used, PGF2α levels increase less rapidly due to inhibition of their synthesis. The duration of pregnancy and delivery will therefore be prolonged in pregnant women taking NSAIDs.

I-8-5. Haematological effects [2,38,51].

Problems with haemostasis are mainly due to acetylsalicylic acid, even at low doses. Cytotoxic accidents are mainly seen with pyrazoles. These may be benign side-effects, detected by haematological tests (anaemia, leucopenia, thrombocytopenia) or serious accidents, which are fortunately rare but often unpredictable, with a sometimes fatal course (haemolytic anaemia, agranulocytosis, bone marrow aplasia, which is fatal in 50% of cases).

I-8-6. Mucocutaneous effects [2,34,52,53].

NSAIDs can cause both allergic and non-allergic hypersensitivity reactions. Allergic reactions are caused by a variety of mechanisms: rarely anaphylaxis, lymphocyte activation or photosensitisation. The latter, which are more common, involve an imbalance in the arachidonic acid degradation pathway. The actual cause is still unknown, but a deficiency in prostaglandin E2, an excess of leukotrienes cysteines, and some genetic polymorphisms have been observed. They can appear in the form of pruritus, urticaria and various rashes, but also rhinitis, bronchospasm and even angioedema or anaphylactic shock. There is also a rare risk of serious dermatitis, such as Lyell's or Stevens-Johnson syndrome. Widal's syndrome has been described as a combination of allergy to acetylsalicylic acid, asthma and nasosinusal polyposis.

I-8-7. Hepatic effects [2,34,54]

These may occur: NSAIDs may be responsible for hepatitis, transient and reversible changes in liver parameters (increase in transaminases, bilirubin). If liver function abnormalities persist or worsen, or if clinical signs of liver failure occur, the NSAID should be discontinued.

I-8-8. Pulmonary effects [2,46,55]

The use of NSAIDs in predisposed patients, such as asthmatics, may exacerbate bronchoconstriction. This undesirable effect is due, on the one hand, to the inhibition of the synthesis of PGE2, a powerful bronchodilator, and, on the other hand, to the orientation of arachidonic acid towards the synthesis of another type of prostanoid with bronchoconstrictor activity.

II- SELF-MEDICATION

II-1. BACKGROUND

Etymologically, self-medication is made up of two words: a prefix "autos" meaning oneself in Greek and "medicatio" meaning the use of a remedy in Latin [56].

According to the WHO, "self-medication is the use of a medicine by an individual, on his or her own initiative or that of a friend or family member, to treat a self-identified condition or symptom, without recourse to a health professional". Self-medication may involve both modern and traditional medicine [10].

The French pharmaceutical industry association for responsible self-medication (AFIPA) has adopted the same definition and added that "reusing a prescribed medicine without the advice of a healthcare professional is not considered responsible self-medication: it is a dangerous practice and contrary to the proper use of healthcare products". [57]. She likens the term "responsible self-medication" to "self-care", which "refers to the individual taking responsibility for his or her own health, including prevention, the environment, a healthy lifestyle, healthy eating and therefore responsible self-medication" [57]. Responsible self-medication implies rational use of the patient's capacity for self-care and excludes practices that are dangerous to health [58-60].

According to the Conseil National de l'Ordre des Médecins (CNOM): Use without a medical prescription by individuals for themselves or for their relatives and on their own initiative, of medicines considered as such and having received marketing authorisation, with the possibility of assistance and advice from pharmacists [61].

The WHO definition can be usefully supplemented by that of the Direction de la Recherche des Études et de l'Évaluation des Statistiques (DRESS) in 2001, which describes the different facets of self-medication: self-medication is a generic term which can describe very different realities. An individual's behaviour when faced with a health problem is self-medication if he or she decides not to seek the advice of a healthcare professional when choosing and following a course of treatment. Treatment is then the sole responsibility of the individual. In practice, any medicine can be used without medical advice, for example by using the medicine cabinet, whether or not the product requires a prescription. Similarly, all medicines can be prescribed by a doctor regardless of the regulatory conditions under which they are dispensed [62].

II-2. PLAYERS IN SELF-MEDICATION

II-2-1. The patient [22,63,64]

They have gradually become active players in their own health and health care, with greater access to information, medical knowledge and even medical expertise in some cases. They are primarily responsible for self-medication. They are the first to identify a symptom or illness and take the initiative to choose a drug themselves, without medical advice, in order to find relief.

II-2-2. The doctor [22,58,63]

The doctor contributes to the patient's overall care ("collaborative care"), with a role of information and advice that goes beyond the limited framework of a prescription or a specific pathology. To ensure maximum patient safety, doctors also have a role to play in monitoring drug consumption, including outside their own prescriptions. This includes the use of self-medication specialities as well as medicines from the medicine cabinet. Patients do not always talk about self-medication, and doctors, often because of time constraints, do not necessarily explain that the medicine should not be taken without medical advice. In fact, the information to be given, specific to the consultation, is often already dense and the addition of a message of prevention on self-medication, in anticipation of a behaviour, seems difficult to achieve. Yet doctors have a duty to inform their patients. This corresponds to their educational obligation to inform patients, and to their responsibility in the field of health. **II-2-3. The pharmacist** [22,58,63,65]

Pharmacists are the only healthcare professionals capable of cross-referencing a patient's medication history or medical condition with the patient's desire to obtain a particular non-prescription medicine. Their close relationship with the patient means that they are in a privileged position to help prevent certain risks to the patient. While one of the pharmacist's roles is to dispense medicines, they have a "*special duty to advise when dispensing medicines that do not require a medical prescription*". Their role in advising, informing and guiding patients makes them one of the pillars of the development of self-medication.

II-2-4. Third-party interveners [25,66,67]

Patients refer a great deal to the experiences of those around them, as well as to other people suffering from the same symptoms. Whether it's a family member or friend, social networks or advertising, they play a significant role in encouraging patients to self-medicate by suggesting therapeutic alternatives.

II-2-5. Pharmaceutical industries [63,68]

Medicines are now promoted through highly sophisticated marketing strategies in which the prescribing doctor is no longer necessarily the central figure. Pharmaceutical advertising is increasingly aimed at the general public, helping to redefine the boundaries of disease and encouraging the medicalisation of everyday life.

II-2-6. Public authorities [69,70]

Self-medication was advocated by the public authorities for economic reasons: to reduce the cost of health insurance and free up doctors' waiting rooms for minor ailments.

II-3. CAUSES OF SELF-MEDICATION [22,25-27,63,69-74]

There are a number of reasons why people turn to self-medication, including their knowledge and perception of the symptoms experienced by the patient. These factors vary according to socio-cultural level, ability to observe, beliefs, education, psychological aspects and advertising. Self-medication can be justified for the following reasons:

■ Knowledge

- ■ Dissatisfaction with the medical profession
- ■ Taking ownership of your illness
- ■ Self-medication as a social phenomenon
- ■ Depression and anxiety
- ■ Easy access to medicines
- ■ Time management
- ■ Economic factors
- ■ Advertising

II-4. SOURCES OF SELF-MEDICATION [18,24,25,75-79]

The main sources of self-medication are :

- ■ Medicines bought over the counter at the pharmacy
- ■ Medicines recommended by the pharmacist
- ■ Medicines prescribed by a doctor, the surplus of which is kept and reused (family pharmacy)
- ■ Medicines provided by family and friends
- ■ Medicines in high-street pharmacies

II-5. RISKS OF SELF-MEDICATION [10,22,69,71,75,79-82].

The risks depend on the drugs used, the patient's co-morbidities, a non-pathological condition requiring special precautions (pregnancy, *etc.*), drug combinations and the duration of self-medication, which can lead to delayed diagnosis. This may result in :

- ■ A self-diagnosis with a high probability of being incorrect.
- ■ Even a correct diagnosis can be followed by an incorrect choice of treatment.
- ■ Consumers will not know whether they belong to a particular group at risk of serious side effects, such as pregnant women, people with weakened immune systems, the elderly, etc.
- ■ The layperson will have no knowledge of the contra-indications, warnings and precautions that can lead to serious side-effects.
- ■ Inability to recognise ongoing adverse reactions
- ■ There is a risk of double medication (if a patient is already taking the same active substance under a different name) or of harmful drug interactions with other medicines taken at the same time.
- ■ Risk of incorrect route/mode of administration of the drug
- ■ Inadequate or excessive dosage with risk of dependence and abuse

■ The risk of shortages of medicines for people who really need them for other illnesses.

■ Storage in incorrect conditions or beyond recommended shelf life

■ Delayed diagnosis of the disease in question, particularly in the case of prolonged self-medication

II-6. ADVANTAGES OF SELF-MEDICATION [57-59,75].

■ It gives patients a sense of responsibility and helps them to take a renewed interest in their health.

■ Rapid management of symptoms.

■ For benign pathologies, this means "less waiting time for GPs, who then have more time to treat patients with serious pathologies requiring regular follow-up".

Chapter 2

Patients and method

1. PATIENTS

I-1. Scope of the study

The rheumatology department of the CHU de Cocody in Abidjan was the setting for our study. It comprises a 26-bed inpatient unit and a consultation unit for diagnosing and monitoring patients. Along with Bouaké, this is the only 2 rheumatology department in Côte d'Ivoire.

I-2. Duration of the study

Patients were recruited over a 6-month period from 1er February 2023 to 31 July 2023.

I-3. Study population

I-3-1. Criteria

We recruited patients meeting the following criteria:

- **Inclusion criteria**
- Any patient with osteoarticular pain who has attended a rheumatology consultation at least once.
- Any patient who has self-medicated with NSAIDs for osteoarticular pain, regardless of the route of administration, duration of use or length of time on the drug.

■ **Non-inclusion criteria**

❖ Any patient who cannot identify the NSAID used.

I-3-2. Sampling

Our minimum sample size was 310. This number

was calculated on the basis of an expected prevalence of 72% (found in a study carried out in Abidjan on the factors determining the consumption of street drugs in urban areas [27]), a confidence interval of 95% and a margin of error of 5%.

The formula used to calculate the sample size was the Swartz formula:

$$N = \frac{z^2}{m^2} * p(1-p)$$

❖ **N** = sample size

❖ **z** = 1.96 for a confidence level of 95%.

❖ **p** = estimated proportion of the population with the characteristic

❖ **m** = 5% margin of error tolerated

$$N = \frac{1{,}96^2}{0{,}05^2} \times 0{,}72\,(1\text{-}0{,}72) = 310$$

II. METHOD

II-1. Type of study

This was a descriptive and analytical cross-sectional study.

II-2. Data collection

Data was collected using a pre-established form.

We looked at the following parameters:

- Socio-demographic data: hospital frequency, age, gender, socio-professional category, marital status, socio-economic level (NSE), level of education and origin;
- Clinical data: patient history, reason for using the AINS, nature of the pain (onset, timing, intensity, location, duration)
- Therapeutic data: drugs (names of molecules, NSAID classes, duration of NSAID use), source of supply, reasons for self-medication, pain results.

II-3. Data analysis

The data were entered and analysed using SPSS version 25 software. A simple description of the sample was possible by calculating proportions and means. The Chi2 test was used to compare proportions and determine the existence of associations between sociodemographic, clinical and therapeutic factors and self-medication. The Fisher test was used when appropriate. The parametric ANOVA test was used to compare the means of quantitative variables in the groups of patients who had or had not self-medicated. The risk of error was set at 5%. The odds ratio (OR) was calculated to determine the relationship between socio demographic and clinical factors and self medication.

For the analytical part, we formed and compared two groups:

- A group of self-medicating patients;
- A control group of patients who had not self-medicated.

We compared socio-demographic and clinical factors between these two groups to identify factors associated with self-medication.

II-4. Ethical considerations

The confidentiality and anonymity of the people surveyed were respected.

II-5. Limits of the study

This work was carried out in the only rheumatology department in Abidjan. Despite the confidential and anonymous nature of the study, it was difficult for us to verify the veracity of the answers provided by the respondents. Although the sample was large, it does not reflect reality in Côte d'Ivoire.

II-6. Operational definitions

- **Professional and managerial staff** are a category of people who have decision-making powers, the ability to conceive and take the initiative. They are required to work even beyond approved working hours, without necessarily expecting remuneration. They are divided into :
- High-level executives: including certain professions such as higher education teachers, administrative executives, doctors, etc.
- Middle management: the people who do the work. They carry out what the above-mentioned people decide. Here, overtime is paid. They include teachers, midwives and secretaries.
- **The informal sector** is a group of activities producing goods and services that are not structured (workers, shopkeepers, farmers, surface technicians, hoteliers, cashiers, shop assistants).
- **Level of education**: refers to the highest level of education achieved by the patient after leaving school.
- Higher level: patients who have continued their education beyond the Baccalauréat.
- Secondary level: those between the 6th and final year of secondary school.
- Primary level: between CP1 and CM2.
- **The socio-economic level (SEL)** was defined arbitrarily on the basis of the guaranteed inter-professional minimum wage (75,000F CFA=115.38 euros).
- Low socio-economic level: if the patient had less than 250,000 F CFA (382 euros) per month
- Average socio-economic level: between 250,000 CFA francs and 500,000 CFA francs (763 euros) per month.
- High socio-economic level: when the patient had more than 500,000 CFA francs per month.
- **Marital status** here referred to a person's marital status. Thus we note :
- Singles: people who live alone and have never been legally married.
- The married: those who are legally united in marriage
- Cohabitees: people who live together as a couple but are not legally married.
- Divorcees: those living alone who have separated from their spouse and broken their marriage contract.
- A widower is someone who lives alone and whose legal spouse has died.
- **Pain intensity** was assessed using a numerical scale from 0 to 10.
- Severe pain corresponded to pain greater than or equal to 7.
- Moderate pain was defined as pain between 4 and 6.
- Mild pain was defined as pain between 1 and 3.

Chapter 3

Results

I. GENERAL DATA
I-1. Socio-demographic characteristics
I-1-1. Hospital frequency
The hospital frequency of self-medication with NSAIDs was 76.67%, i.e. 388 out of
506 patients recruited during the study period.
I-1-2. Age

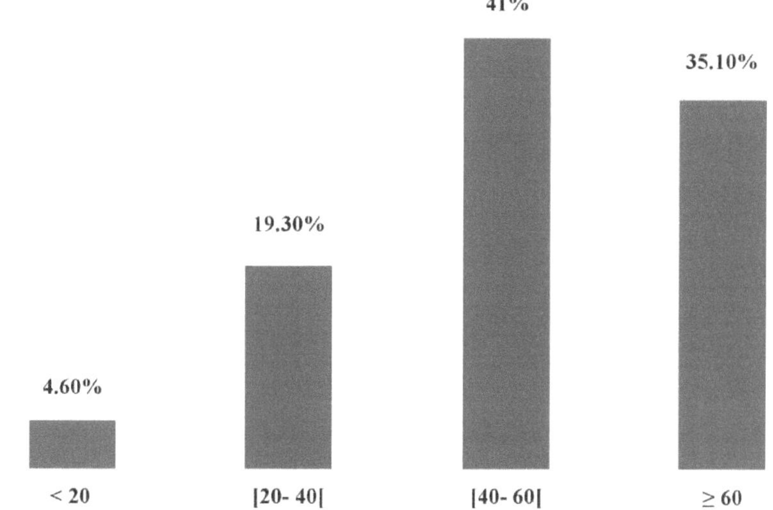

Figure 2: Breakdown of patients by age group

The dominant age group was 40 years and over (76.10%).
Average age: 52 +/- 16 years [extremes: 8 and 84 years].
I-1-3. Type

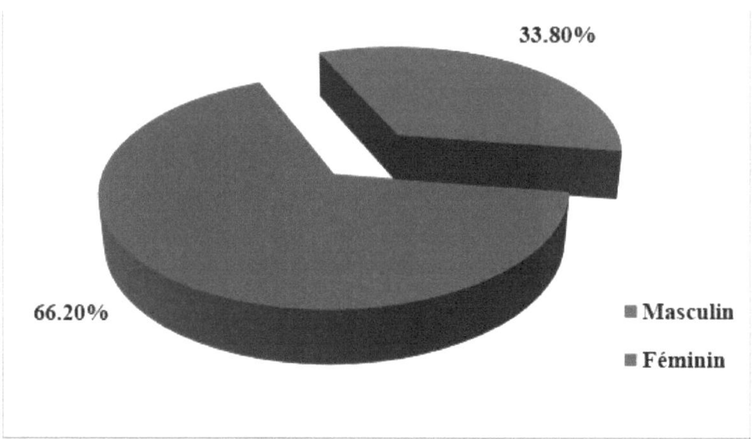

Figure 3: Breakdown of patients by gender

Females predominated (66.20%), with a sex ratio (M/F) of 0.51.

I-1-4. Marital status

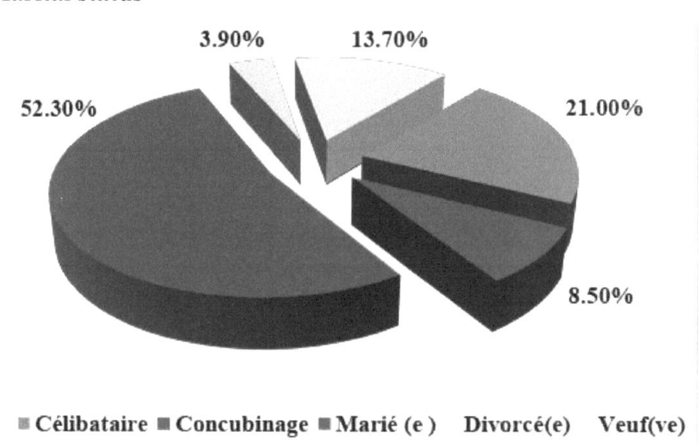

Figure 4: Breakdown of patients by marital status
Just over half the patients were married (52.30%).

I-1-5. Socio-economic level (NSE)

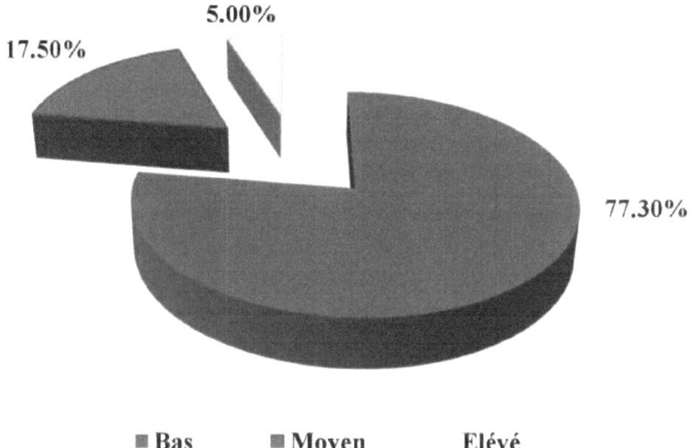

Figure 5: Breakdown of patients by socio-economic status

The majority of patients had a low ESN (77.30%).

I-1-6. Level of study

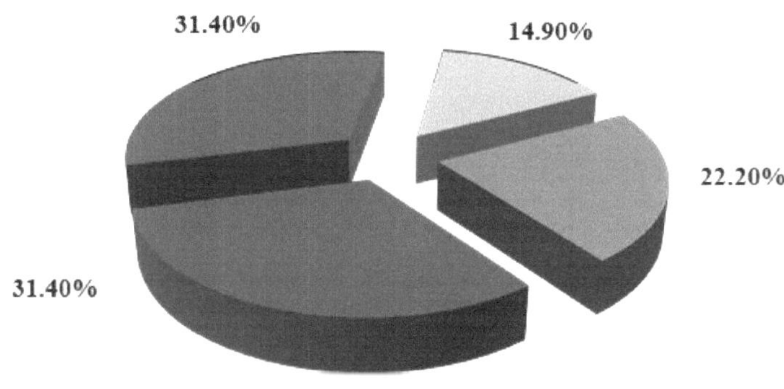

Figure 6: Breakdown of patients by level of education

Patients attending school accounted for 85.10% of our patient population.

I-1-7. Source

Table VI: Breakdown of patients by region of origin

Area of origin	Workforce		Percentage
Rural areas	43	11,1	
Urban area	**345**	**88,9**	
Total	388	100	

The majority of our patients lived in urban areas (88.9%).

I-1-8. Socioprofessional categories

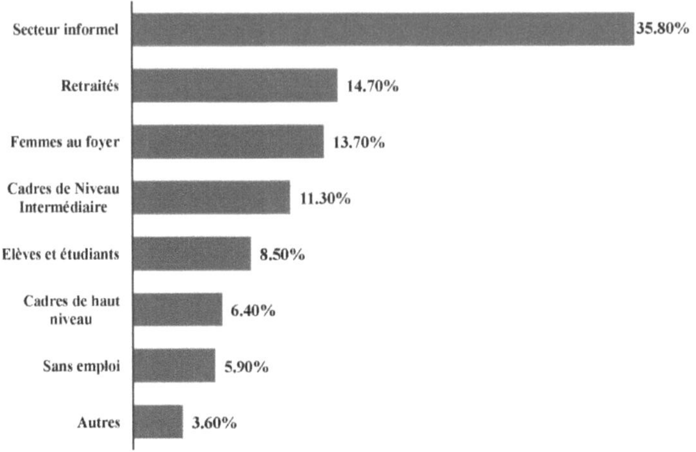

Figure 7: Breakdown of patients by socio-professional category

The dominant socio-professional category was in the informal sector (35.80%).

I-2. Clinical characteristics

I-2-1. Background

Table VII: Breakdown of patients by comorbidity

Comorbidities	Workforce	Percentage
HTA	**100**	**25,77**
UGD	**58**	**14,94**
Diabetes	38	9,8
Infections	14	3,6
Sickle cell disease	5	1,3

The main comorbidities were hypertension (25.77%) and peptic ulcer disease (14.90%).

I-2-2. Reasons for using NSAIDs

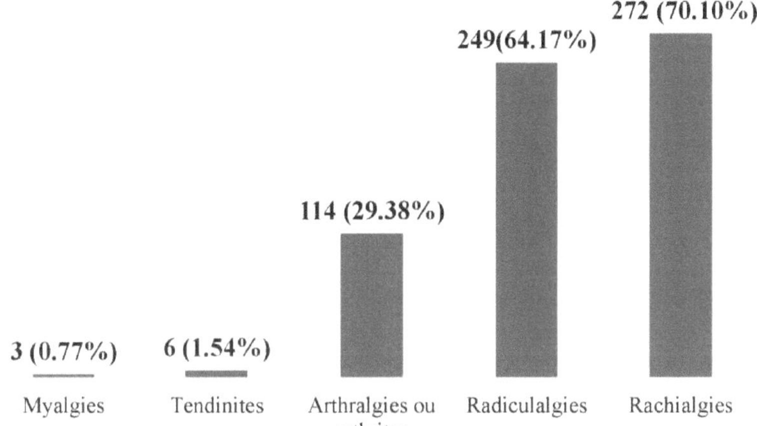

Figure 8: Breakdown of patients by reason for NSAID use

Most NSAIDs were used for spinal pain (70.10%) and spinal pain with radiculalgia (64.17%).

I-2-2-1. Different locations of spinal pain

Table VIII: Breakdown of patients by location of spinal pain

Spinal pain	Workforce	Percentage
Neck pain	21	7,70
Back pain	61	22,40
Low back pain	**236**	**86,80**
Fessalgia	01	0,40

Low back pain was the most common spinal pain (86.80%).

I-2-3. Character of the pain

I-2-3-1. Timetable

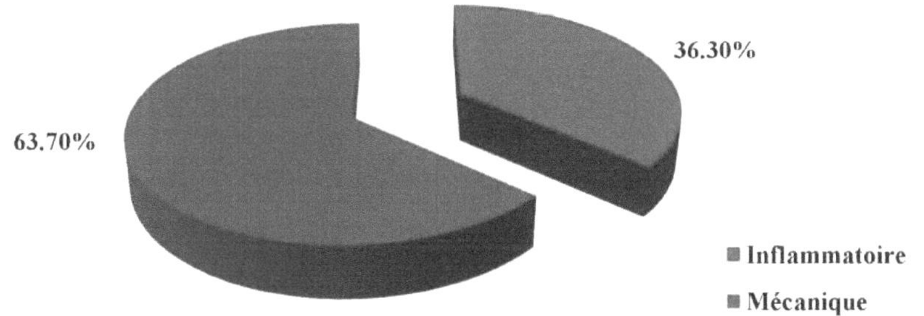

Figure 9: Breakdown by pain schedule

Mechanical pain predominated (63.70%).

I-2-3-2. Start mode

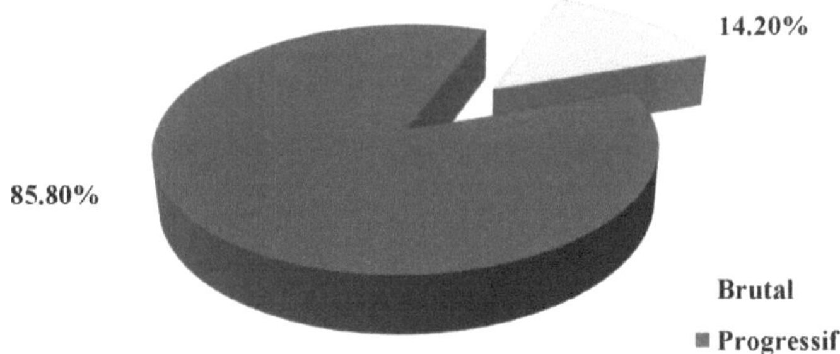

Figure 10: Breakdown by pain onset mode

Pain set in gradually in the majority of cases (85.80%).

I-2-3-3. Seat

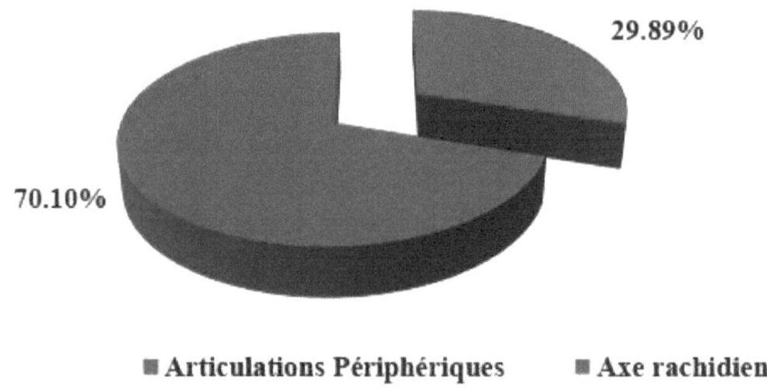

Figure 11: Distribution according to site of pain Most of the pain was axial (70.10%).

I-2-3-4. Development time

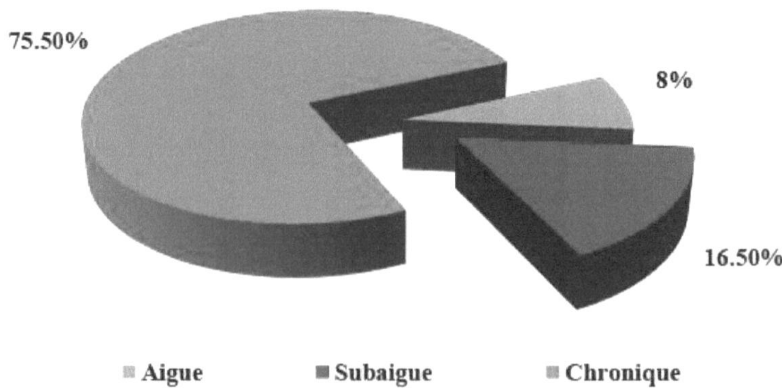

Figure 12: Breakdown by duration of symptoms

The majority of patients had symptoms lasting more than three months (75.50%).

I-2-3-5. Pain intensity

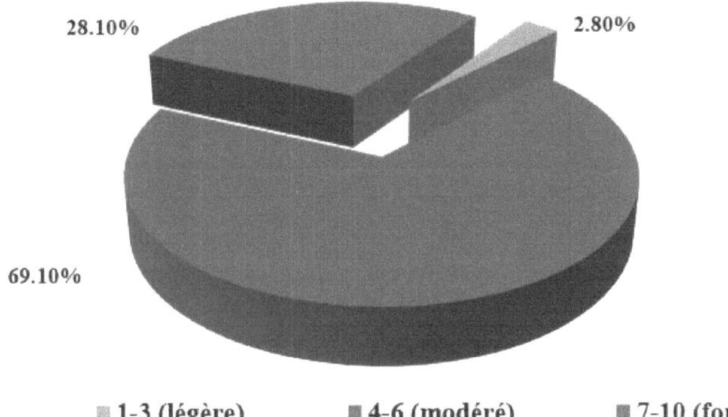

Figure 13: Distribution according to pain intensity The majority of patients had pain of moderate intensity (69.10%).
).

I-3. Therapeutic characteristics

I-3-1. Type of NSAIDs used

Table IX: Breakdown by class of NSAIDs used

Therapeutic class	Workforce	Percentage
Arylcarboxylic	**346**	**89,2**
Oxicams	26	6,7
Fenamates	08	2,1
Coxibs	26	6,7
Salicylic	01	0,3

The most commonly used NSAIDs belonged to the arylcarboxylic family (89.2%).

I-3-2. Molecules of NSAIDs consumed

Table X: Breakdown by NSAID molecule used

	Workforce	Percentage
Diclofenac	**296**	**76,28**
Ibuprofen	46	11,85
Aceclofenac	29	7,47
Ketoprofene	29	7,47
Piroxicam	30	7,70
Niflumic acid	08	2,06
Etoricoxib	14	3,60

| Celecoxib | 12 | 3,09 |
| Acetylsalicylic acid | 01 | 0,25 |

The most commonly used NSAID was diclofenac (76.28%).

I-3-3. Duration of consumption of NSAIDs

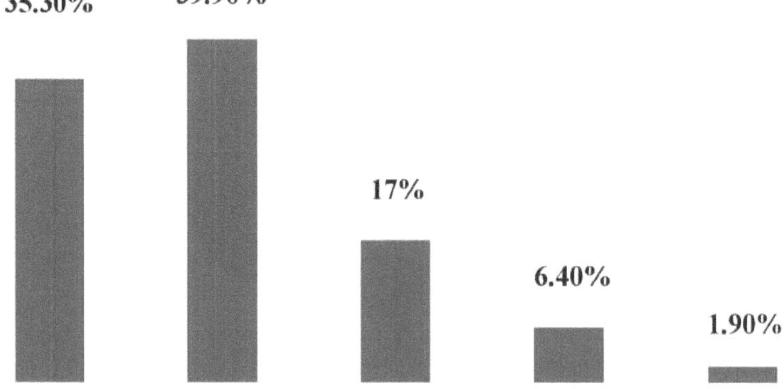

Figure 14: **Breakdown by duration of NSAID use**

The majority of NSAIDs were taken between 1 and 13 days (75.20%).

I-3-4. Place of supply of NSAIDs

Tableau XI: Breakdown by place of supply of NSAIDs

Supply location	Workforce	Percentage
Pharmacy	**295**	**76**
Rue	200	51,5
Third party	36	9,3
Family pharmacy	38	9,8

Pharmacies (76%) and the street (51.5%) were the main sources of NSAIDs.

I-3-5. Reasons for self-medication

Tableau XII: Breakdown by reason for self-medication

	Workforce		Percentage
Accessibility (space and time)	**259**	**66,85**	
Third-party advice	**205**	**52,83**	
Effective based on previous experience	165		42,5
Lack of financial resources	143	36,85	
Dispensing without a prescription	112		28,9
Retail sales	24		6,2
Identical to those sold in pharmacies	14		3,6

The reasons given by patients for self-medication were accessibility (66.85%) and advice from a third party (52.83%).

<u>**Tableau XIII:**</u>   Breakdown by source of advice on self-medication

	Workforce	Percentage
Friends	**133**	**64,87**
Advertising	42	20,48
Family	30	14,63

The majority of people were influenced by friends (64.87%).

I-3-6. Effectiveness on pain

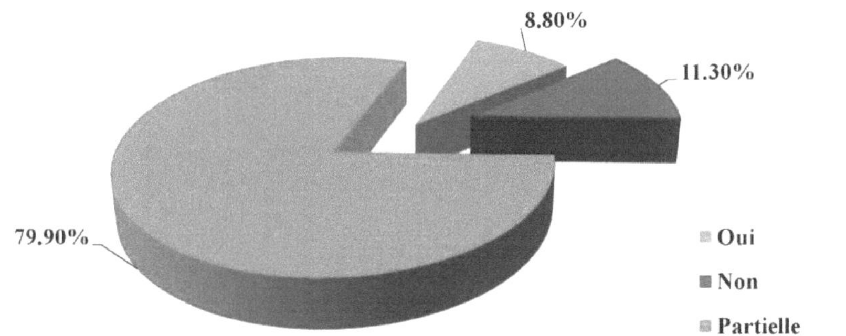

<u>Figure 15</u> : Distribution according to the effectiveness of NSAIDs on pain

Self-medication with NSAIDs was only partially effective in reducing pain in the majority of patients (79.90%).

I-3-7. Satisfaction

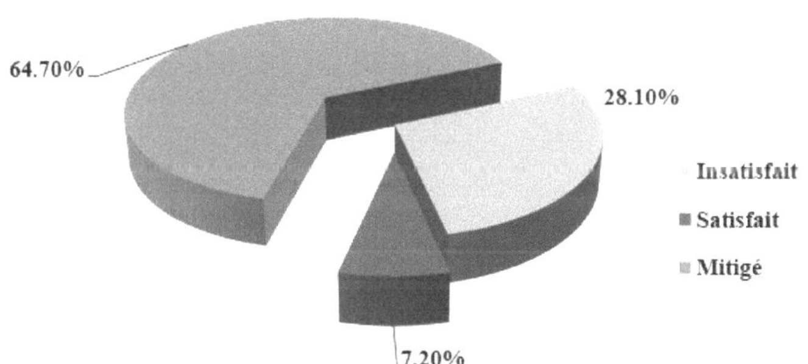

<u>Figure 16:</u> Distribution according to patient satisfaction after taking NSAIDs

More than half the patients had mixed satisfaction after taking NSAIDs.

I-3-8. Patients' assessment of their self-medication

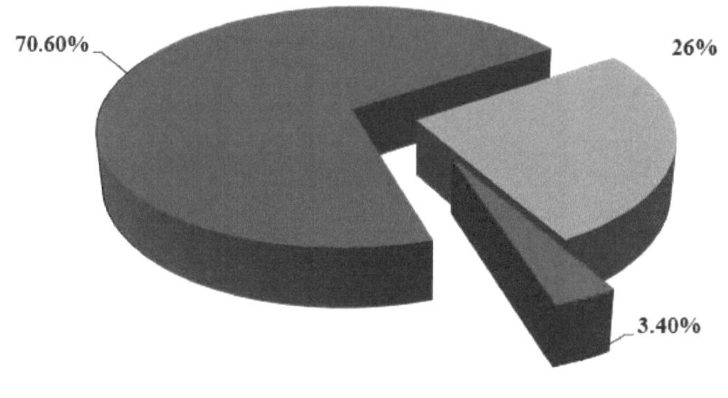

Figure 17: Breakdown of patients' views on self-medication

Most patients thought their attitudes were wrong.

II-ANALYTICAL DATA

II-1. Socio-demographic characteristics

Table XIV: Association between sociodemographic factors and self-medication

Socio-demographic factors	Self-medication (+)	Self-medication (-)	OR (95% CI)	P
Average age	52 ±16	53±14,7		0,341
GenderMale	131	33		0,143
Female	257	85		
Level of study				
Schoolchildren	330	95	1,109	**0,046**
Not enrolled	58	23	(1,026-1,348)	
Marital status				
Single	84	24		
Cohabitation	33	7		0,823
Divorced	15	5		
Married	203	62		
Widowed	53	20		
Source				
Rural	43	10		0,267
Urban	345	108		
Socio-economic level economic				
Low	300	97	1,158	**0,039**
Medium/educated	88	21	(1,052-1,543)	

(+): Presence   (-): Absence

Level of education and socio-economic status were significantly associated with self-medication, with p-values of 0.046 and 0.039 respectively.

II-2. Clinical characteristics

<u>**Table XV**</u>: Association between pain characteristics and self-medication

Type of pain	Self-medication (+)	Self-medication (-)	OR	P
Timetable				
Mechanical engineering	247	80		0,239
Inflammatory	141	38		
Start mode				
Brutal	55	17		0,308
Progressive	333	46		
Evolution				
Sharp	31	12		
Subaigue	64	20		0,751
Chronicle	293	86		
Intensity				
Slight	11	8	1,448	**0,011**
Moderate	268	83	(1,184-2,207)	
Severe	109	27		

Pain intensity was significantly associated with self-medication.

Chapter 4

Discussion

I-1. SOCIO-DEMOGRAPHIC CHARACTERISTICS

■ The hospital incidence of self-medication with NSAIDs was 76.67%, or 388 out of 506 patients recruited during the study period. These results were consistent with those reported in the literature from sub-Saharan Africa, North Africa, Asia and Oceania, where the figures ranged from 59% to 81.8% [19,23,24,27,83-86]. However, in some sub-Saharan African studies, the proportions were significantly lower than ours, particularly in Burkina Faso (52.60%) and Cameroon (37.5%) [80,87]. This difference with the Burkina Faso and Cameroon studies could be explained by the fact that they were based solely on pharmacies and did not take into account street medicines or those available at hand, which are a major source of supply for self-medication. According to the World Bank, in 2015, more than half of the poor lived in sub-Saharan Africa, and more than 85% in sub-Saharan Africa and South Asia [88]. This could explain their low capacity to seek care, and therefore very low levels of effective and appropriate healthcare spending. The decision to consult a doctor as soon as a symptom appears is largely dependent on the financial resources available. Added to this are inequalities in health and access to care, which remain considerable. One of the main consequences of this lack of access to healthcare is the reluctance to go to health centres as a first line of defence. It seems very easy to take the step of self-medicating with NSAIDs when faced with pain that is causing discomfort, especially as the NSAID will be used to soothe the pain.

■ The dominant age group was 40 years and over (76.10%) with a mean age of 52 +/- 16 years, which was close to the figures of Nessib et al in Tunisia (56 years) [67]. In most African and Asian studies, young adults were found, with ages ranging from 33 to 42.4 years.
[19,24,26,83,89,90]. In Europe, particularly in France, the subjects were elderly (62 years) [91]. This variation could be explained by the youth of the African population and the ageing population in the West [92,93]. This may explain why there was no significant association between age and self-medication in our study.

■ There was a predominance of women (66.20%) with a sex ratio (M/F) of 0.51. This predominance had also been found in several studies [26,53,63,66,69,75,76,85,90,94-96]. There could be several reasons for this predominance among women: the pain is thought to result from the various daily gestures and postures of women, who are the housekeepers. They are housewives and work in the informal sector, which involves prolonged inappropriate postures that cause pain. NSAIDs are more readily available than going to a health centre, sometimes to save time. Women also have a lower pain threshold than men, which explains why women make much greater use of medication than men for the same amount of pain [97,98]. This inequality between the sexes is thought to be underpinned by hormonal factors: testosterone is thought to reduce excitatory nociceptive activity, whereas oestrogen and progesterone (the dominant hormones in women) are thought to have a pronociceptive effect by reducing the inhibitory component of pain [97,98]. However, our study showed no link between gender and self-medication.

■ The majority of our patients attended school (85.10%). The same observation has been made in the literature, with rates of up to 100% depending on the study [19,22-24,66,75,83,89,90,96]. It seemed paradoxical that patients with a good level of education should resort to self-medication. These apparently well-educated patients gave themselves the right to treat themselves even though they did not belong to the medical profession. Is it pride or laziness in honouring a consultation? Added to this is the information available and accessible on social networks, the media and the internet. Hence the significant association between level of education and self-medication in our study.

■ The socio-economic level was low in the majority of our patients (77.30%) as in the literature with Shafi et al in Ethiopia (60%), Abdelmoneim et al in Sudan (74.20%), Angbo-Effi et al in Côte d'Ivoire (85.18%), Gupta et al in India (91.3%) and could be linked to the modest economic conditions of most of our patients as in most sub-Saharan countries [23,24,27,95]. Self-medication offers a "false" cheap alternative to people who cannot afford a consultation. As a result, it is often the first response to illness among people on low incomes. In our study, there was a significant association between socio-economic level and self-medication.

■ Just over half the patients were married (52.30%). Our data were close to those of Sallam et al in Egypt (61.7%), Shafi et al in Ethiopia (67.5%), Divya et al in India (73%) [24,83,90]. However, they were higher than those of Gobir et al in Nigeria, Ndol et al in the DRC, Makita-Ikouaya et al in Gabon, and Al-

Ghamdi et al in Saudi Arabia, who found 44%, 40.6%, 22% and 24.8% respectively [19,26,85,89]. In our study, marital status was not significantly associated with self-medication.

■ The majority socio-professional category was in the informal sector (35.80%). The same finding was made by Ouané in Mali (32.8%), Souaga et al in Côte d'Ivoire (33.33%), Gobir et al in Nigeria (39.6%), Hamani in Niger (70%) [28,89,99,100]. In developing countries, the economy is dominated by the informal sector, which employs a large proportion of the population. It is a sector of activity that is insufficiently structured, in which workers live on what they earn on a daily basis. It is in this sector that street medicines develop more easily. NSAIDs are accessible and available over the counter. This is what we call "the pharmacy on the ground", and the epicentre of this pharmacy is the large market in Adjamé, where there is a dedicated area (the area around the former Roxy cinema). Everyone can obtain NSAIDs very easily. However, socio-professional category was not linked to self-medication in our study.

■ The majority of our patients lived in urban areas (88.9%), as was the case in several studies [24,69,78]. This could be explained by the concentration of medical facilities in urban areas. Urban areas are where over-the-counter and retail NSAIDs are sold.

I-2. CLINICAL CHARACTERISTICS

■ Hypertension and peptic ulcer were the main comorbidities found in the patients in our study, in 25.77% and 14.90% of cases respectively. This is consistent with the results of Guilliano in Haiti, who found hypertension (7.9%) and peptic ulcer disease (9.9%) to be the main comorbidities [76]. Ouedraogo et al in Burkina Faso found peptic ulcer to be the main comorbidity, but in lower proportions than ours (7%) [20]. The difference in proportions can be explained not only by the larger sample size in our study, but also by the fact that the study population was self-medicated exclusively with NSAIDs. Peptic ulcer disease is the most frequent side effect of NSAIDs (except coxibs), with proven digestive toxicity [2,101,102]. The older the patient, the more harmful the toxicity. Epidemiological studies have consistently shown that the risk of digestive complications increases with age (symptomatic ulcers, haemorrhage, perforation, stenosis). This increase with age may be linked to reduced resistance of the gastroduodenal mucosa to aggression, changes in the pharmacokinetics of NSAIDs (physiological ageing modifies the distribution, metabolism and elimination of NSAIDs) and polypathology [102-104].

With regard to hypertension, in addition to the other causes of hypertension in patients, it should be noted that numerous studies have shown that NSAIDs induce an increase in blood pressure of around 4 mm Hg [105,106]. The increase in blood pressure is generally very moderate in normotensive patients (1 to 2 mm Hg) and greater in hypertensive patients (> 3 mm Hg) [107]. Furthermore, the use of NSAIDs increases the relative risk of developing hypertension by a factor of 1.4 [108]. However, the effects of NSAIDs on blood pressure depend on the type of antihypertensive treatment used [109,110].

■ Most NSAIDs were used for spinal pain (70.10%) and spinal pain with radiculalgia (63.40%). Low back pain was the most common spinal pain (86.8%). Low back pain was also the 1er reason for self-medication with NSAIDs for osteoarticular pain, but in lower proportions in Guilliano (17.2%), Sinclair et al (24.8%), Sivry (37.12%), Ouédraeogo et al (37.37%) and Anger (40.3%) [20,63,75,76,94]. Spinal pain is the most frequent reason for consultation in rheumatology practice, particularly low back pain [111,112]. The lumbar region is a mobile area and is therefore subject to high levels of daily mechanical stress, which could wear away the functional unit of the lumbar spine, whose elastic properties diminish during the ageing process.

■ The majority of patients had symptoms lasting more than three months (75.5%), as in the study by Sinclair et al in Scotland, but in a lower proportion (37.5%) [94]. This could be explained by the trivialisation of symptoms that can be temporarily alleviated by NSAIDs. There was no statistically significant association between duration of symptomatology and self-medication.

■ In our study, the majority of patients had pain of moderate intensity (69.10%). Chindhalore et al in India, and Ouedraeogo et al in Burkina Faso, reported a majority of patients with pain of severe intensity, respectively 45% and 57.6% of cases [20,113]. This could be explained by the fact that most rheumatic diseases are progressive in onset and generally better tolerated. Pain intensity was associated with self-medication in our study.

I-3. THERAPEUTIC CHARACTERISTICS

■ Diclofenac was the most commonly used NSAID in our study (76.28%), as in the studies by Ndol et al in the DRC and Keltoum et al in Algeria [19,22]. A study carried out in our context in 2013 by Diomandé et al showed that ketoprofen dominated at that time [114]. This would prove that the consumption preference for NSAIDs has shifted from ketoprofen to diclofenac in 10 years in Côte d'Ivoire. In Asia, diclofenac also dominated, as did South America with 14% and 22% respectively [113,115]. In the West, ibuprofen occupied 1st place [53,63,116]. This difference may be explained by the wide availability and accessibility of diclofenac both in pharmacies and in "pharmacies on the street". It is the best-known NSAID in our context, is widely prescribed by nursing staff and has the highest proportion of generic drugs.

■ In terms of duration of use, the majority of NSAIDs were taken between 7 and 13 days (39.90%), in contrast to the literature where NSAIDs were almost all taken between 1 and 6 days [63,76,116]. This difference may be explained by the particular nature of our study population. These were middle-aged rheumatic patients, most of whom suffered from pain related to daily mechanical and occupational stress, in contrast to other studies in which NSAIDs were used for a variety of occasional complaints such as dysmenorrhoea, headache and flu-like symptoms.

■ Pharmacies (76%) and the street (51.5%) were the main sources of NSAIDs. This was found in several African and Asian studies [17,18,117,20-22,24,28,53,76,84]. In European studies, dispensaries or family pharmacies were the main sources of supply [63,75]. In developing countries, legislation on the sale of medicinal substances is not respected, and the sale of medicines on the sly on the streets, in markets and on buses is common, with the risk of using counterfeit, out-of-date or poorly preserved medicines.

■ Accessibility (poor reception by nursing staff, long waiting times, insufficient staff), advice from a third party, efficacy based on previous experience and lack of financial resources were the main reasons given by patients for self-medication in 66.8%, 52.83%, 42.5% and 36.85% of cases respectively. These data are consistent with the literature [20,22,24,28,63,76,83,84,86,90,115,117]. In Africa, community life is very strong, which could explain the influence of friends and family in self-medication. The majority of the population have a low socio-economic level and take refuge in self-medication to avoid spending money in health facilities. Also, patients, who for the most part live and support their families on what they earn on a daily basis, and faced with long queues for consultations and an insufficient number of doctors, resort to an individual solution in order to save time.

■ In our study, most patients thought that their attitudes were bad (70.6%). This was also found by Ouedraogo et al (89.9%), Fuentes et al (77%), Keltoum (77%) [20,22,115]. Although they were aware of this, they chose to self-medicate in the face of socio-economic realities. This attitude therefore appeared to be resignation on the part of these patients.

Conclusion

The frequency of self-medication with NSAIDs is very high in Abidjan. Women of mature age, with a high level of education, low socio-economic status and working in the informal sector are affected. Self-medicated NSAIDs are used for chronic mechanical spinal pain with a gradual onset. Accessibility and advice from a third party are the main reasons for self-medication with NSAIDs, the most commonly used of which belong to the arylcarboxylic family, led by diclofenac, which is taken for less than two weeks. Patients buy their NSAIDs in pharmacies and on the street, but they are only partially effective in relieving pain, giving mixed satisfaction and rating their self-medication as bad. The factors determining consumption were level of education, socio-economic status and pain intensity.

Based on our findings, we make the following recommendations to :

- **Political decision-makers**

- Intensify controls to stop the parallel market in NSAIDs on the street.

- Dismantling the large "Roxy" market in Adjamé

- Intensify mass education on the dangers of self-medication with NSAIDs, with the participation of medical learned societies.

- Applying the regulations governing the sale of NSAIDs in pharmacies.

- **Doctors**

- Take the time to educate their patients about the practice of self-medication, and advise against taking any medicines without consulting a doctor.

- Fill prescriptions correctly, limiting the number of days they can be used.

- **Pharmacists**

- Do not prescribe NSAIDs.

- Do not renew an NSAID prescription without your doctor's advice.

- **Patients**

- Always consult a doctor in the event of symptoms.

- Always take NSAIDs on medical advice.

- Follow the instructions on the prescription.

References

1. **Blain H, Jouzeau JY, Netter P, Jeandel C**. Les anti-inflammatoires non steroidiens inhibiteurs selectifs de la cyclooxygenase 2. Interest and prospects. Rev Med Interne 2000;21(11):978-88.

2. **Wirth H, Hürlimann R, Flückiger T**. NSAIDs and COX-2 inhibitors: main adverse effects. Forum Médical Suisse 2006;6(12):284- 90.

3. **Lévy P, Fanello S, Pivette J, Parot-Schinkel E, Le Grand G, Schoux JB, Le Bodo P**. Non-steroidal anti-inflammatory drugs and potential iatrogenic risks: analysis of health insurance data. Rev Med Assur Mal 2005;36(2):153-62.

4. **Doomra R, Goyal A**. Universal health coverage - there is more to it than meets the eye. J Family Med Prim Care 2017;6(2):169-70.

5. **Da Silva ER, De Rose EH, Ribeiro JP, Sampedro LBR, Devos DV, Ferreira AO, Kruel1 M**. Non-steroidal anti-inflammatory use in the XV Pan-American Games (2007). Br J Sports Med 2011;45(2): 91- 4.

6. **Gorski T, Cadore LE, Santana PS, Marczwski DSE, Silva Correa C, Beltrami GF**. Use of NSAIDs in triathletes: prevalence, level of awareness and reasons for use. Br J Sports Med 2011; 45(2):85-90.

7. **Koffeman AR, Valkhoff VE, Celik S, Jong GW, Sturkenboom MC, Bindels PJE, et al**. High-risk use of over-the-counter non-steroidal anti-inflammatory drugs: a population-based cross-sectional study. Br J Gen Pract 2014; 64(621):191-8.

8. **Didier S, Vauthier JC, Gambier N, Renaud P, Chenuel B, Poussel M**. Substance use and misuse in a mountain ultramarathon: new insight into ultrarunners population? Res Sport Med 2017;25(2):244-51.

9. French National Agency for the Safety of Medicines (ANSM). Reminder of the rules for the proper use of non steroidal anti inflammatory drugs (NSAIDs). European Journal of Emergency and Intensive Care 2013; 25(3-4):197-200.

10. World health Organization (WHO). Guidelines for the regulatory assessment of medicinal products for use in self medication. Geneva: WHO; 2000: 30p.

11. **Albasheer OB, Mahfouz MS, Masmali BM, Ageeli RA, Majrashi AM, Hakami AN**. Self-medication practice among undergraduate medical students of a Saudi tertiary institution. Trop J Pharm Res 2016 ;15(10):2253-9.

12. **Rashid M, Chhabra M, Kashyap A, Undela K, Gudi SK**. Prevalence and predictors of self-medication practices in India: a systematic literature review and meta-analysis. Curr Clin Pharmacol 2020;15(2):90-101.

13. **Wijesinghe P, Jayakody R, Seneviratne R**. Prevalence and predictors of selfmedication in a selected urban and rural district of Sri Lanka. WHO South-East Asia J Public Heal 2012;1(1): 28-41.

14. **Gore PR, Madhavan S**. Consumers preference and willingness to pay for pharmacist counselling for non-prescription medicines. J Clin Pharm Ther 1994;19(1):17-25.

15. **Pfaffenbach G, Tourinho F, Bucaretchi F**. Self-medication among children and adolescents. Curr Drug Saf 2010;5(4):324-8.

16. **Kshirsagar NA**. Rational use of medicines: cost consideration & way forward. Indian J Med Res 2016;144(4):502-5.

17. **Jaleta A, Tesema S, Yimam B.** Self-medication practice in Sire town, west Ethiopia: a cross-sectional study. Cukurova Med J 2016;41(3):447-52.

18. **Osemene KP, Lamikanra A**. A study of the prevalence of self-medication practice among university students in southwestern Nigeria. Trop J Pharm Res 2012;11(4):683-9.

19. **Ndol FMI, Bompeka FL, Dramaix-Wilmet M, Meert P, Malengreau M, Mangani NN, et al**. Self-medication among patients admitted to the emergency department of Kinshasa university hospital. Santé Publique 2013;25(2):233-40.

20. **Ouédraogo D, Tiendrebeogo JWZ, Zongo E, Kakpovi KG, Kaboré F, Drabo JY, et al.** Prevalence and factors associated with self-medication in rheumatology in Sub-Saharan Africa. Eur J Rheumatol 2015;2(2): 52-6.

21. **Ocan M, Bwanga F, Bbosa GS, Bagenda D, Waako P, Ogwal- J et al**. Patterns and predictors of self-medication in northern Uganda. PLoS One 2014; 9 (3) : 1-7.

22. **Keltoum T, Amina N**. Self-medication with non-steroidal anti-inflammatory drugs. Mémoire Med. Guelma: Université 8 Mai 1945; 2021: 95p.

23. **Awad AI, Eltayeb IB, Capps PA**. Self-medication practices in Khartoum State, Sudan. Eur J Clin Pharmacol 2006;62(4):317-24.

24. **Shafie M, Eyasu M, Muzeyin K, Worku Y, Martín-Aragón S**. Prevalence and determinants of self-medication practice among selected households in Addis Ababa community. PLoS One 2018;13(3):1-20.

25. **Raynaud D**. Determinants of self-medication. Rev Fr Aff Soc 2008;1:81-94.

26. **Makita-ikouaya E**. Determinants of the use of self-medication among patients living in the commune of libreville (Gabon). Revue de Géographie Tropicale et d'Environnement 2020;1:148-58.

27. **Angbo-Effi KO, Kouassi DP, Yao GHA, Douba A, Secki R, Kadjo A**. Factors determining the consumption of street medicines in urban areas. Santé Publique 2011;23(6):455-64.

28. **Souaga K, Adou A, Amantchi D, Kouame P, Angoh Y**. Self-medication for oral diseases in urban Côte d'Ivoire. Results of a survey in the Abidjan region. Odontostomatol Trop 2000;23(90):29-34.

29. **Hounsa A, Kouadio PDM**. Self-medication with antibiotics from private

pharmacies in the city of Abidjan, Côte d'Ivoire. Med Mal Infect 2010;40:333-40.

30. **Orliaguet G, Gall O, Benabess-lambert F**. New developments in steroidal and non-steroidal anti-inflammatory drugs. Le Praticien en Anesthesie Réanimation 2013;17(5):228-37.

31. **Viel E, Ripart J EJ**. Pharmacology of non-steroidal anti-inflammatory drugs and indications for postoperative analgesia. In: Blanloeil Y. Conférences d'actualisation 2000. Paris: Masson. 2000;323-34.

32. Sociéte Francaise de Rhumatologie (SFR). Anti-inflammatory drugs. Available at: https://public.larhumatologie. fr/les-anti-inflammatoires (consulted on 15/07/23)

33. **Tréchot P, Jouzeau JY**. Chemical and pharmacological bases of NSAIDs. Rev Fr Allergol 2014;54(3):212-7.

34. **Marotte H**. French College of Teachers of Rheumatology (COFER). 6th ed. Paris: Masson; 2018: 433p.

35. **Badou M, Bertin P**. Non-steroidal anti-inflammatory drugs: prescription and monitoring. In: Faillie JC, Perrot S. Le bon usage du médicament et des thérapeutiques non médicamenteuses. 5eme ed. Paris : Medline ; 2012 : 337-48.

36. **Mazières B.** Les Anti-inflammatoires non stéroidiens. In: Laroche M, Mazières B, Constantin A, Cantagrel A. Rhumatologie pour le praticien. Paris: Masson; 2018: 619-36.

37. **Dorosz P, Vital Durand CLJ**. Practical guide to DOROSZ medicines. 29ème ed. Paris: Maloine; 2009: 2048p.

38. **Levet E**. Non-steroidal anti-inflammatory drugs: risk factors for worsening bacterial infections. Pharmacists' knowledge of this potential risk. Thèse Pharm. Limoges : Univ Limoges ; 2011 : 89p.

39. **Timour Q, Bui-Xuan B**. Subjects at physiological risk: age, pregnancy and breastfeeding. Paris: EMC Odontologie; 2008.

40. **Charles Caulin**. Le dictionnaire vidal. 86ème ed. Paris: Vidal; 2010: 3000p.

41. Reference centre for teratogenic agents. Non-steroidal anti-inflammatory drugs and pregnancy. Available at: http://www.lecrat.org/article.php3?id_article=649 (consulted on 17/07/23)

42. **Laharie D, Droz-Perroteau C, Bénichou J, Amouretti M, Blin P, Bégaud B, et al**. Hospitalizations for gastrointestinal and cardiovascular events in the CADEUS cohort of traditional or Coxib NSAID users. Br J Clin Pharmacol 2010;69(3):295-302.

43. **Wallace JL**. Mechanisms, prevention and clinical implications of nonsteroidal anti-inflammatory drug-enteropathy. World J Gastroenterol 2013;19(12): 1861-76.

44. **Masso Gonzalez EL, Patrignani P, Tacconelli S GR LA.** Variability among nonsteroidal anti-inflammatory drugs in risk of upper gastrointestinal bleeding. Arthritis Rheum 2010;62(6):1592-601.

45. **Strate LL, Liu YL, Huang ES, Giovannucci EL, Chan AT**. Use of aspirin or nonsteroidal anti-inflammatory drugs increases risk for diverticulitis and diverticular bleeding. Gastroenterology 2011;140(5):1427-33.

46. **Emer M, Burke A, Garret A, FitzGerald**. Lipid-derived autacoids: eicosanoids and platelet-activating factor. In: Laurence L. Brunton. The pharmacological basis of therapeutics. 11th ed. California: Mcgraw-Hill Medical Publishing Division; 2006: 653-70.

47. **Adam WR**. Non-steroidal anti-inflammatory drugs and the risks of acute renal failure: Number needed to harm. Nephrology 2011;16(2):154-5.

48. **Bentley ML, Corwin HL, Dasta J**. Drug-induced acute kidney injury in the critically ill adult: Recognition and prevention strategies. Crit Care Med 2010;38(6):169-174.

49. **Lafrance JP**. Selective and non-selective non-steroidal anti-inflammatory drugs and the risk of acute kidney injury. Pharmacoepidemiol Drug Saf 2009;7:923 -31.

50. **Soubrier M, Rosenbaum D, Tatar Z, Lahaye C, Dubost JJ, Mathieu S.** Nonsteroidal anti-inflammatory agents and vessels. Rev Rhum 2013;80(3):204 - 8.

51. **Benoit A**. Non-steroidal anti-inflammatory drugs and risk of infection: regional survey of dispensing pharmacists and pharmacy students. Thèse Pharm. Bourgogne : Univ Bourgogne; 2020 : 123p.

52. **Demoly P.** Les hypersensibilités aux anti-inflammatoires non stédroidiens, anciens et nouveaux concepts. Which explorations? Revue Française d'Allergologie et d'Immunologie Clinique 2007;47:60-2.

53. **None R**. Adverse effects of non-steroidal anti-inflammatory drugs and Self-medication: what is the impact over time of a written information tool on patients' knowledge? Thèse Med. Bourgogne : Univ Bourgogne; 2017 : 73p.

54. **Vuillet-A-Ciles H, Buxeraud J, Nouaille Y**. Pain medications: tier I analgesics. Actual Pharm 2013;52(527):21-6.

55. **Daham K, Song WL, Lawson JA, Kupczyk M, Gülich A, Dahlén SE et al.** Effects of celecoxib on major prostaglandins in asthma. Clin Exp Allergy 2011;41(1):36-45.

56. Self-medication. Dictionary of the French National Academy of Pharmacy. Available at: http://dictionnaire.acadpharm.org/w/Automédication (consulted on 16/07/23)

57. AFIPA. Definition of responsible self-medication. 2010; available at

https://sante. gouv. fr/IMG/pdf/Contribution_de_l_AFIPA.pdf (consulted on 16/07/23)

58. **Coulomb A, Baumelou A.** Situation de l'automédication en France et perspectives d'évolution : marché, comportements, positions des acteurs. Paris: La Documentation Française; 2007: 31p.

59. **Fainzang S**. L'automédication, une pratique qui peut en cacher une autre. Anthropol Sociétés 2010;34(1):115-33.

60. **Baumelou A.** Self-medication and public health. Bull Acad Natle Med 2007; 191(8):1527-31.

61. **Pouillard J**. Self-medication. Rapport adopté lors de la session du Conseil national de l'Ordre des médecins. Paris: CNOM; 2001: 7p.

62. **Parrot J**. From self-diagnosis to self-medication: risks and impact on the pharmacist-patient relationship. Bull Acad Natle Med 2007;191(8):1509-15.

63. **Sivry P**. Self-medication of non-steroidal anti-inflammatory drugs - evaluation of the level of knowledge of 334 patients in general practices in the Alpes-Maritimes. Thèse Med. Nice : Univ Nice Sophia-antipolis; 2014 : 66p.

64. **Degos L**. Automédication: le patient acteur de sa santé. Bull Acad Natl Med 2007;191(8):1503-8.

65. **Chaspierre A**. A front-line health player? Santé conjuguée 2011; 55:84-8.

66. **Lecocq-Verdin AL**. Self-medication with NSAIDs: advantages and disadvantages. Thèse Pharm. Rouen: Univ Rouen; 2014. 174p.

67. **Nessib BD, Benbrahim A, Maatallah K, Ferjani H, Triki W, Kaffel WH**. Self-medication in rheumatology: prevalence and associated factors. Rev Rhum 2021;88(1): A299.

68. **Cathébras P**. Le docteur Knock habite à Wall Street: Les nouvelles cibles de l'industrie pharmaceutique. Rev Med Interne 2003;24(8):538-41.

69. **Hmaini N**. L'automedication et la medication officinale : Enquete par questionnaire dans les pharmacies de la province de khemisset. Thèse Med. Rabat : Univ Mohammed V; 2017 : 150p.

70. **Seddik M, Yahia B**. Epidemiological survey on self-medication in the wilaya of Jijel. Mémoire Med. Jijel: Univ Mohammed Seddik Ben Yahia; 2019 : 83p.

71. **Montastruc JL, Bondon-guittona E, Abadie D, Lacroix I, Sailler L, Damase-michel C**. Pharmacovigilance: risks and adverse effects of self-medication. Revue Thérapie 2016;71(2): 249-55.

72. **Sridhar SB, Shariff A, Dallah L, Anas D.** Assessment of nature, reasons and consequences of self-medication practice among general population of Ras Al- Khaimah, UAE. Int J Appl Basic Med Res 2018;8(1): 3-8.

73. **Kassabi-Borowiec L, Lévy P**. Factors and modalities of self-medication in

general practice. Lettr Pharmacol 2002;16(2): 61-3.

74. **Klohn M VI**. Self-medication. Med Mal Infect 2008;40(6):333-40.

75. **Anger V**. Self-medication with non-steroidal anti-inflammatory drugs (NSAIDs): a review of knowledge and patient practices in the Somme in 2018. Thèse Med. Amiens: Univ Picardie Jules Verne; 2019: 68p.

76. **Guilliano A**. Survey on the knowledge of non-steroidal anti-inflammatory drugs consumed in self-medication conducted among 203 patients received at the general consultation service of the Haiti State University Hospital during the month of September 2019. Thesis Med. Port-au-Prince : Univ Haïti ; 2020 : 69p.

77. **Rouanet C**. Self-medication in pharmacies in Antananarivo (Madagascar). Thèse Pharm. Lyon : Univ Claude Bernard Lyon 1; 2018 : 112p.

78. **Faqihi SF**. Self-medication practice with analgesics (NSAIDs and acetaminophen) and antibiotics among nursing undergraduates in university college Farasan campus, Jazan University, KSA. Ann Pharm Fr 2021;79(3):275-81.

79. **Ray I, Bardhan M, Mehedi M, Moiz A, Khan E, Patel S et al**. Over the counter drugs and self-medication: A worldwide paranoia and a troublesome situation in India during the COVID-19 pandemic. Ann Med Surg 2022;78(1):103.

80. **Lassana S**. Self-medication in the city of Ouagadougou: a survey of pharmacies. Thèse Pharm. Ouagadougou: Université de Ouagadougou;1999: 111p.

81. **Queneau P**. Débat: l'automédication, source de dangers? Bull. Acad. Natle Med 2007;191(8): 1535-37.

82. **Queneau P, Bannwarth B**. Adverse drug reactions observed in French reception and emergency departments. Bull Acad Natl Med 2003;187(4):647-70.

83. **Sallam SA, Khallafallah NM, Ibrahim NK, Okasha AO**. Pharmacoepidemiological study of self-medication in adults attending pharmacies in Alexandria, Egypt. East Mediterr Heal J 2009;15(3):683-91.

84. **Phalke V, Phalke B, Durgawale M**. Self-medication practices in rural Maharashtra. Indian J Community Med 2006;31(1):35-6.

85. **Al-Ghamdi S, Alfauri TM, Alharbi MA, Alsaihati MM, Alshaykh MM, Alharbi AA et al**. Current self-medication practices in the kingdom of Saudi Arabia: An observational study. Pan Afr Med J 2020;37(51):1-16.

86. **Ngo SNT, Stupans I, Leong WS, Osman M**. Appropriate use of non-prescription ibuprofen: a survey of patients perceptions and understanding. Int J Pharm Pract 2010;18(1):63-5.

87. **Loe GE, Ngoule CC, Ngene JP, Pouka MP**. Evaluation of self-medication

with analgesics in adults: the case of customers of dispensing pharmacies in Douala, Cameroon. Int J Biol Chem Sci 2017;11(4):1461-70.

88. **Dean J, Lugo M**. Poverty and shared prosperity 2018. Washington: World bank Group; 2018. 201 p.

89. **Gobir A., M. N. Sambo SSB**. Assessment of pattern of non-steroidal antiInflammatory drugs (NSAIDS) use among residents of a north central nigerian city. Trop J Heal Sci 2017;24(4):1-6.

90. **Divya M, Bharatesh S, Vasudeva G**. Self-medication among adults in urban Udupi Taluk, Southern India. Int J Med Public Heal 2016;6(3):126-9.

91. **Hesberta A, Louisa V, Curisb E, Briotc K, Gossecc L, Poireaudeaud S, et al**. Self-medication in rheumatology. Pharm Hosp Clin 2012 ;47:S11-S95.

92. **Michele Dion M**. Ageing. L'Europe en Formation 2015; 3 (377): 46-60.

93. <u>Economic Commission for Africa. Demographic profile of Africa.</u> Addis Ababa: UNFPA; 2016: 1-78.

94. **Sinclair HK, Bond CM, Hannaford PC**. Over-the-counter ibuprofen: how and why is it used? Int J Pharm Pract 2000;8(2):121-7.

95. **Gupta P, Bobhate PS, Shrivastava SR**. Determinants of self medication practices in an urban slum community. Asian J Pharm Clin Res 2011;4(3):54-7.

96. **Matoulkova P, Dosedel M, Ruzková B, Kubena** A. Information and awareness concerning ibuprofen as an ingredient in over the counter analgesics: A questionnaire-based survey of residents of retirement communities. Acta Pol Pharm 2013;70(2):333-8.

97. **Gaumond I, Marchand S**. L'inégalité des sexes dans la douleur : un mythe devenu réalité. Douleurs Evaluation-Diagnostic-Traitement 2009;10(5):230-6.

98. **Javier RM PS**. Are men and women different when it comes to pain? What impact does this have on the rheumatologist's practice? Rev Rhum 2010;77:227-9.

99. **Ouane M**. Analyse de la dispensation des anti-inflammatoires en milieu officinal à Bamako: cas de 30 officines. Thèse Med. Bamako: Univ Bamako; 2004: 77p.

100. **Hamani A**. Les médicaments de la rue à Niamey: Modalités de vente et contrôle de qualité de quelques médicaments anti-infectieux. Thèse Med. Bamako: Univ Bamako; 2005: 140p.

101. **Wallace JL**. Prostaglandins, NSAIDS, and gastric mucosal protection: why doesn't the stomach digest itself? Physiol Rev 2008;88:1547-65.

102. **Bannwarth B.** Les antalgiques et anti-inflammatoires non stéroïdien chez le sujet âgé. Rev Rhum 2004;71:534-8.

103. **Verlhac B.** Non-steroidal anti-inflammatory drugs in the elderly and iatrogenic accidents: the most important points. Rev Rhum

2004;71:S179-S82.

104. **Legrain S.** Prescription médicamenteuse du sujet âgé. Paris: EMC Médecine; 2005.

105. **Chrischilles E.** Nonsteroidal anti-inflammatory drugs and blood pressure in an elderly population. J Gerontol 1993;48:M91-6.

106. **Johnson G, Nguyen T.** Do non-steroidal anti-inflammatory drugs affect blood pressure? A meta-analysis. Ann Intern Med 1994;121:289-300.

107. Effect of stepped care treatment on the incidence of myocardial infarction and angina pectoris: 5-year findings of the hypertension detection and follow-up programme. Hypertension 1984 ; 6 (2) :I198-206.

108. **Pope J, Anderson D.** A meta-analysis on the effect of nonsteroidal antiinflammatory drugs on blood pressure. Arch Intern Med 1993;153:477-84.

109. **Morgan T, Anderson A.** Effect of indomethacin on blood pressure in ederly people with essential hypertension well controlled on amlodipine or enalapril. Am J Hypertens 2000;i3:1161-7.

110. **Le Lorier J, Bombardier C, Burgess E, Moist L, Wright NK C.** Practical considerations for the use of non-steroidal antiinflammatory drugs and cycto- oxygenase-2 inhibitors in hypertension and kidney disease. Can J Cardiol 2002;18:1301-8.

111. **Diomandé M, Bamba A, Traoré A, Kpami Y, Coulibaly Y, Coulibaly A, Djaha M, Gbané M, Ouattara B, Daboiko JC, Eti E.** Epidemiological data on rheumatological hospitalisation in Abidjan (Côte d'Ivoire). Revue Africaine de Médecine Interne 2020;7(1-2):22-30.

112. **Koffi-Tessio V, Oniankitan S, Hé C, Atake A, Kakpovi K, Yibe F, Mba E, Fianyo E, Houzou P, Oniankitan O, Mijiyawa M.** Epidemiological and clinical profile of patients undergoing rheumatological consultations at the Sylvanus Olympio University Hospital.
(Lomé-Togo). Rhum Afr Franc 2021; 4 (1): 1 - 6.

113. **Chindhalore CA, Dakhale GN Giradkar AB.** Comparison of self-medication practices with analgesics among undergraduate medical and paramedical students of a tertiary care questionnaire - based study. J Educ Health Promot 2020;9:309.

114. **Diomandé M, Ouali B, Eti E, Kouakou ESCL, Brou K, Gbané M Djaha M, Ouattara B, Kouakou MN.** Indications, efficacy and tolerance of non-steroidal anti-inflammatory drugs: about 602 prescriptions in the rheumatology department of the CHU Cocody d'Abidjan. Rev Cames Santé 2013;1(2): 93-8.

115. **Fuentes K, Zapata, Lorenzo V.** Analysis and quantification of selfmedication patterns of customers in community pharmacies in southern

Chile. Pharm World Sci 2008;30:863-8.

116. **Nunes AP, Costa IM, Costa FA**. Determinants of self-medication with NSAIDs in a Portuguese community pharmacy. Pharmacy Practice 2016;14(1):1-9.

117. **Suleman S, Ketsela A, Mekonnen Z**. Assessment of self-medication practices in Assendabo town, Jimma zone, southwestern Ethiopia. Res Soc Adm Pharm 2009;5(1):76-81.

Appendix: survey form

Factors determining self-medication with NSAIDs in rheumatology patients in Abidjan

I. Identity and general information

N°

1. Age

2. **Sex**: *Female Male...*

3. **Socio-economic level**: Low (< 250,000 Fcfa) ... Medium (250.000500.000 Fcfa) . High (> 500.000 Fcfa) .

4. **Marital status**: *Single   Married   Widowed...*
Divorced.. Cohabiting.

5. **Socio-professional category**: Pupils and students . Housewife.
Unemployed..   Informal sector. Senior executives.
level ...Mid-level executive ... Retired.
Other

6. **Origin**: Urban Rural

7. **Nationality**: Ivorian. Foreign... (ECOWAS. Outside ECOWAS... Other...)

8. **Ethnic group** :   (Akan.. Gour... North Mande... South Mande...
Krou..)

9. **Level of education**: Not enrolledEducated   (primary)
Secondary University)

II. History

>   Diabete HTA UGD

Heart disease ...   Infections ...

>   Other

III. Reasons for using NSAIDs

>   Spinal pain... (neck pain... spinal pain... low back pain... ear pain...
radiculalgia .)

>   Peripheral joints: arthralgia...   arthritis...

>   Tendonitis ...   Myalgia.

>   Others.

IV. Type of pain

1. **Schedule**: Inflammatory... Mechanical.

2. **Start-up mode:** brutal,   progressive.

3. **Head office :** Axe.. Ring road...

4. **Progression time (Months)** Acute.. Subacute.. Chronic..

5. **Intensity:**   1-3 (light).. 4-6 (moderate).. ≥ 7 (strong)

V. Consumption of NSAIDs

A. **Self-medication:** Yes... No...

1. **If yes :**

a. **Knowledge of NSAIDs**

-   Name the molecules consumed:

-   **Type of NSAID used (INN)**

Carboxylic aryl: Oxicams: Indolics:Fenamates:

Coxib: Salicylates : Sulfonalidine :   Pyrazoles :

b. **Reasons**

Dispensing without a prescription. Previous experience. Lack of financial resources.

Sold in detail . Accessibility (space and time) . Identical to those sold in pharmacies.

Others.

c. **Influence of a third party**

1. Yes... No...

          1. a If yes (FriendsAdvertisingOther   )

d. **Consumption time**

1-6 days: .... 7-13 days: 14 days - 29 days:

30-90 days:..> 90 days : .

e. **Where do you get NSAIDs?**

Pharmacy.   street. Third party. Present within reach.

VI. Results on pain

1. Effectiveness: yes   no   partial

2. if not, what do you decide to do

VII. Satisfaction

Satisfied   Mitigated   Dissatisfied

VIII. What do you think of your attitude?

Good   Wrong   Half good, half bad.

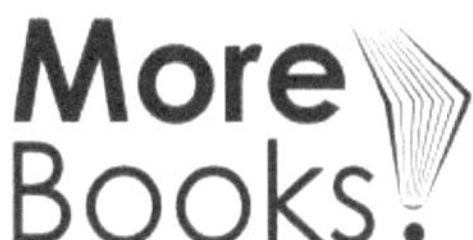
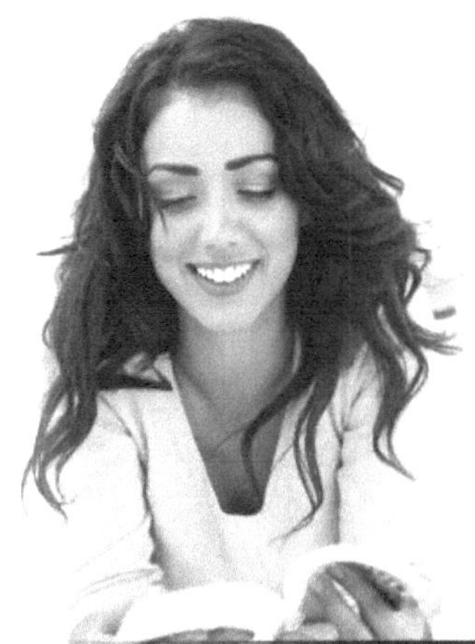

I want morebooks!

Buy your books fast and straightforward online - at one of world's fastest growing online book stores! Environmentally sound due to Print-on-Demand technologies.

Buy your books online at
www.morebooks.shop

Kaufen Sie Ihre Bücher schnell und unkompliziert online – auf einer der am schnellsten wachsenden Buchhandelsplattformen weltweit! Dank Print-On-Demand umwelt- und ressourcenschonend produziert.

Bücher schneller online kaufen
www.morebooks.shop

info@omniscriptum.com
www.omniscriptum.com

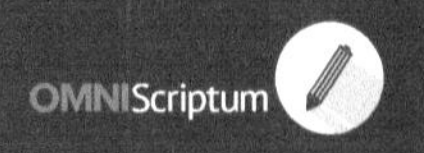

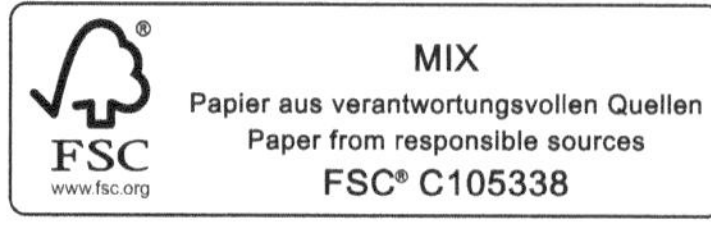

Printed by Books on Demand GmbH, Norderstedt / Germany